100 YEARS OF INSULIN

S. K. SINHA

100 Years of Insulin

S K Sinha

ISBN: 978-0-6489470-2-8 (paperback)
ISBN: 978-0-6489470-3-5 (eBook)

Cover Design: Insulin crystals. Artist's impression. Lee Sinha. © 2022

To my wife Lee

CONTENTS

PREFACE

The story of insulin portrays a triumph of hope over experience.

2021 is remembered as the centenary of the discovery of insulin and 2022 marks one hundred years of the use of insulin in the treatment of patients with diabetes.*

This is the story of that discovery which saved the lives of thousands of children and adults around the world and today enables millions of children and adults to lead normal lives.

This book celebrates the 100th anniversary of the discovery of insulin. It also describes some of the remarkable developments in the knowledge of insulin over the one hundred years since its isolation by an inexperienced medical graduate assisted by an equally inexperienced university student.

A brief description of diabetes would place in perspective the role played by insulin.

Diabetes results from a deficiency of insulin which is a hormone produced in the Islets of Langerhans. The islets are nests of cells found in the pancreas, an organ which produces digestive juices

---

* There is an increasing, and entirely appropriate, appreciation of the necessity to recognise the individual as a person. None of us is defined by an isolated characteristic such as creed, colour or a medical condition. Therefore I have avoided the term "diabetic" except in quotations and seek the reader's forbearance for any oversight in this matter.

needed to break down and digest food. Insulin is needed for taking glucose from the bloodstream (into which it has been released by the Islets of Langerhans) to muscles, fat and the liver where the body produces energy for physical activities and also stores glucose as fat.

There are two kinds of diabetes usually referred to as Type One or Juvenile Diabetes and Type Two, also known as Adult-onset Diabetes. Although insulin is often used in adults with adult–onset or Type Two diabetes its most dramatic effects are seen in Type One diabetes especially in children.

Many articles in the lay and scientific journals reported the discovery in 1921. In 1962 Gerald Wrenshall, Geza Hetenyi, and William R. Feasby published a book, "The Story of Insulin: Forty Years of Success against Diabetes."

In 1971 The Canadian Diabetes Association also produced a popular monograph on insulin by Bernard Leibell and Gerald Wrenshall.

An earlier article published in 1954 by Joseph Hersey Pratt (1872–1956), a Harvard professor who had a lifelong interest in diabetes and who had reviewed the accounts of the discovery of insulin in Toronto, had drawn attention to improvements by Collip in the pancreatic extract produced by Banting and Best. Pratt was persuaded to tone down his article in case it was used to detract from the credit being given to Banting and Best. One of the more vociferous Canadian critics of Pratt's article was W.R. Feasby, a medical historian and an admirer of Charles Best. (Feasby later started on a biography of Charles Best but died before completing it.)

Two books have been written on the discovery of insulin. Just over 60 years after the discovery a Canadian historian called Michael Bliss wrote *The Discovery of Insulin* which was issued forty years ago in 1982. Nearly 20 years were to elapse before a second work, *Margaret and Charlie* written by Henry B.M. Best, a son of Charles Best, was released in 2003. A substantial part of the book was devoted to the discovery of insulin.

Each one of these accounts is presented here in order to provide a background for revisiting the momentous events in Toronto in the two summers of 1921 and 1922 which captured the imagination of millions of men, women and children who suffer from diabetes and offered hope to their families as well as the medical and scientific community throughout the world.

In 1982 the Canadian historian Michael Bliss (1947–2017) published *"The Discovery of Insulin."* Unlike many books on medical subjects which are written by doctors, Bliss presented the account from a layman's point of view which was a refreshing change. His descriptions, and attention to detail through meticulous research including face – to – face interviews, produced an account which read like a detective story. Not afraid to call "a spade a spade," he didn't shy away from providing a "warts and all" narrative of the different characters in the drama of the research which culminated in the discovery. He also provided interesting details of the background of some of the controversies which followed in the wake of the discovery, not the least being the awarding of the Nobel Prize to two of the four participants in the research. More than one of them claimed to be worthy of receiving the prize either for himself or jointly with others.

Bliss, who came from a medical family – his father was a general practitioner and his brother a physiologist – had to overcome many difficulties sifting opinion from fact in the numerous articles in professional and lay journals. Different laboratories reported findings which were often contradictory and a challenge to those in the medical profession let alone a historian like Bliss.

Little wonder then that, perhaps in exasperation, at the very outset of his book he stated: "My aim was to carry out the historian's job of re-creating the discovery of insulin. As far as possible I wanted to work from contemporary sources. I wanted to ignore the judgement of later writers and put aside the partisan recollections of the discoverers themselves, at least until I had found out from the documents generated at the time – laboratory notebooks, correspondence, published articles, etc – exactly what had happened. *I wanted to reconstruct the insulin research dog by dog, day by day, and experiment by experiment.* After that it will be proper to reflect on the fallibility of the participants' memories and the validity of the scientists' claims and counter-claims."

(Italics by the writer).

To call Bliss's plan ambitious would be an understatement. There are many areas in which a man with no experience or background in scientific studies, let alone experimental work, would face significant challenges. Physiology is the study of the way in which different parts (organs) of the body function normally. When the study involves abnormal function it is called pathology. Both physiology and pathology are often referred to as "secondary" subjects because they require basic knowledge of anatomy, or study of the normal body (in men and animals like the dogs used in the research studies carried out in Toronto). Anatomy is taught in the early years of the medical course before exposure to physiology and pathology in the third and fourth years of a six – year course.

A layman would have faced significant hurdles understanding the research without a background in the knowledge of these basic sciences. An added issue for Bliss would have been to follow medical jargon. Making allowances for, let alone explaining, medical, anatomical, physiological and biochemical terms to an outsider especially one with the hunger for details which Bliss certainly had, would not normally be part of a bench scientist's brief.

Bliss's brother James Bliss was a physiologist and a professor of physiology at McGill University. More importantly from the point of view of the insulin project, he was experienced in medical research having carried out experiments on tissue and organ transplants. Unfortunately James Bliss had died in 1969 at the age of 39, some 13 years before his younger brother embarked on his writing project on insulin.

In the introduction to his book Bliss said, "This would have been much better book if he had lived to help write it."

That Michael Bliss was able to overcome so many challenges and succeeded is a testament to his tenacity and scholarship. *The Discovery of Insulin* published in 1982 is probably the most widely read book on this topic.

Margaret and Charley the Personal Story of Dr. Charles Best, the Co-Discoverer of Insulin.

Henry B.M. Best.

"They set out to preserve and inform."

In 2003 Charles Best's son Henry Bruce Macleod Best wrote *Margaret and Charley. The Personal Story of Dr. Charles Best, the Co-Discoverer of Insulin.* Most of the material contained in this 500-page book is drawn from the papers and letters from the remarkable collection which his parents had kept throughout their lives perhaps with the aim of writing a joint-biography. Unfortunately this did not occur.

Henry Best (1937–2006) was Charles Best's younger son. He had taught Canadian history at York University and had served as President of Laurentian University. It is clear from reading the book that Charles Best and his wife Margaret Mahon Best were not only devoted to one another but were also avid letter writers and, Margaret Best in particular, kept detailed records, letters and diary notes throughout their marriage of more than 50 years.

In the introduction to his book, Henry Best says, "the role of the historian in making scientific judgements, or judgements about scientists, is a fascinating one. Historians assess politicians, soldiers, churchmen, and many others, so why not scientists? One reply is that we should not judge those whose lives have been of note in such fields without relevant preparation in their particular profession. If this view were followed, many historians would be out of business."

The book by Henry Best contains details of the insulin story as recorded by Charles Best himself or by Margaret Mahon Best, the writer's wife. Particularly useful for my purposes were Charles Best's letters to his wife which, unlike scientific information, were written from the heart. They were his personal impressions of various people who played a part in the discovery of insulin. These make interesting reading even if some facts or opinions could be challenged by others. Best, at the time of his involvement with work on insulin was simply a medical student looking for a job during the summer to provide him with pocket money. He had attended lectures on carbohydrates which had been delivered by the Head of the department, Professor James Macleod. Macleod was an academic who had written a book on carbohydrate metabolism but had had pursued an academic career. There is no record of him ever being involved in the medical care of diabetics in any capacity. Best had had limited laboratory experience. His book-knowledge of diabetes had come from lectures at the university. There was no reason to devote extra time to diabetes or, for that matter, to any particular medical condition in a course on physiology which is a study of *normal* workings of different systems in the human body.

I was conscious of the personal nature of the information in Henry Best's book. Differences between Charles Best's opinions and comments from the views of outsiders must be interpreted in the light of his writings being intended for his family records and not necessarily for publication or for examination by those outside his family.

It is important that his views on the controversy regarding the Nobel Prize awarded in 1923 be interpreted in the context of his age and experience at that time. At the time of the discovery he was only 22 years old.

Henry Best's book was published in 2003 when he was 66 years old. With few exceptions, he wrote from the material in the Best family archives. It is fascinating to read of his very restrained assessment of his father's efforts in various areas of academic and social activities. For example, very early in his reading of the family archives, he realised that his father had recognised the value of "networking" before the term had come into common use.

I sensed his patience and generosity when making that judgement on his father who at that time was in his early 20s because Henry Best at the time of writing *Margaret and Charley* was in his 60s with a lifetime of experience in academia as well as in public and political life.

In spite of the obvious differences the two works are complementary. Bliss's book strives for objectivity while Henry Best steers clear of expressing his own views and simply relates the information found in his parents' voluminous material. However Best the history professor, could not resist the temptation of joining in the Nobel Prize controversy. One could graciously ascribe this to family loyalty but some, after reading this book, may choose to differ.

My interest in diabetes began when I started as an intern following my graduation from the medical school at the University of Sydney, Australia and continued throughout the forty years of my professional life as a physician/internist specialising in the treatment of diabetes.

Good teachers can change lives.

During a Fellowship at the Joslin Diabetes Centre during the early years of my postgraduate education I had the advantage of working with a group of remarkable men and women who had devoted their lives to the treatment of diabetes.

My own journey of discovery in the field of diabetes owes a great deal to men and women whose guidance and personalities influenced my thinking and professional development especially my interest and involvement in the treatment of children and adults with diabetes.

Remaining in contact with such teachers amongst the physicians of the Joslin Diabetes Centre in Boston following my years as a Fellow in 1969 and 1970 has been an influence on my thoughts on clinical medicine, medical research as well as medical history.

Dr Priscilla White and Dr Alexander Marble had been with Dr Joslin at the time of the introduction of insulin in the treatment of diabetes. Joslin's practice was one of the first in the United States to be given a supply of the extracts of insulin largely because of the large number of patients with diabetes in his practice but also because of his close association with the discoverers of insulin, Banting and Best.

I had the privilege of working with Dr. Priscilla White during the summer of 1970, when I had the responsibility of managing the Clara Barton summer camp for girls with diabetes. This gave me an insight not only into the finer points of the treatment of diabetes but also the rare opportunity of getting to know a truly remarkable physician. Several of the friendships which began in Boston have been an important part of my life and a source of inspiration even after my retirement from active practice.

The discovery of insulin was, and still is, highlighted in chapters devoted to the history of diabetes in medical textbooks. However a comprehensive account suitable for the general public has not been written in recent years.

This work revisits the story of that discovery and traces the progress and research in several fields in the second half of the twentieth century which have culminated in unlocking the mystery of the insulin molecule. As a result of these advances, now for the first time, "modern" insulin production is no longer dependent on animal sources.

By providing a sequel to the exciting discovery in 1921, this book brings the reader to the present day in the knowledge of and information on the fascinating, life-saving and life-changing hormone called insulin.

Shailendra K. Sinha
Sydney
Australia.
2022

INTRODUCTION

INSULIN A DAILY MIRACLE FOR MILLIONS

"It was as simple as this: insulin worked wonders, near–miracles, time after time."
Michael Bliss in *The Discovery of Insulin* 1982.

"Yet, can the reader imagine the feelings of a doctor with a background of 1000 fatal cases, who has lived to see what the ages have longed for come true in the discovery of insulin....."
Elliott Proctor Joslin, *Treatment of Diabetes Mellitus*. Third Edition. 1923.

"It still remains a wonder, that this limpid liquid injected under the skin twice a day can metamorphose a frail baby, child, adult, or old man or woman to their nearly normal counterparts."
Elliott Proctor Joslin 1923.

This is the story of insulin, a miracle which is remembered each and every day by millions around the world.

Insulin was discovered in 1921 in a small city in Canada. At the time Canada was not a leader in medical science let alone in medical research. The discovery brought world-wide fame and prominence not only to Toronto, where the laboratories were housed, but also to the entire country of Canada.

That single event in the summer of 1921 changed the fate of countless children and adults around the world. It happened during a period in human history when diabetes claimed lives of children as young as two years. Young men and women ravaged by the disease were reduced to states of unspeakable debility. Some likened them to prisoners of Concentration Camps of the Second World War.

The discovery of insulin in the summer of 1921 turned a fatal ailment into a manageable condition and allowed thousands to live beyond their normal life expectancy. Today nearly 500 million adults and more than 1 million children and adolescents are living with diabetes. Virtually all the children and many of the adults depend on receiving insulin every day for survival.

This story speaks of the heartaches of parents who watched helplessly as their children suffered and were then lifted into the realm of hope even optimism that insulin held the promise of an end to their sense of helplessness and hopelessness.

There have been other miracles.

Antibiotics allowed man to conquer infective illnesses like scarlet fever, yellow fever and tuberculosis. But they're not a part of everyday living.

Unlike other great discoveries of medications which have saved lives when needed, the millions of men, women and children who depend on daily injections of insulin are reminded of its life-changing effect *every day*.

Diabetes does not respect geography or race. Insulin is used by children, young people and adults in isolated habitats, in mountain villages. Natives in the depths of the tropical jungles in Africa and South America use it. In the midst of many a thriving metropolis in first world countries the restorative properties of insulin are relied upon every day just as they are in the small islands of the archipelagoes in the Pacific Ocean.

Insulin made it possible for those suffering from diabetes to control the level of glucose in their blood. It gave them the freedom to go about their daily lives with little disruption. Indeed unless they chose to speak of the condition, one would have been hard pressed to detect any difference between them and their friends, colleagues, and even their relatives. Dramatic changes made as a result of progress in the development of insulin, it's method of delivery as well as technological advances in many related areas of medical practice paint a very different picture of the care of children and adults with diabetes today.

But it was not always like this.

A brief account of the condition of many affected individuals before the discovery of insulin may place in perspective the extraordinary sense of anticipation at the very first indication of the possibility, no matter how tenuous, of relief let alone the possibility of many patients' lives being spared.

Today's individual with diabetes would hardly recognise one suffering from this condition 100 years ago. On average, a child with diabetes usually did not survive more than three years. The afflicted children were in many instances, barely conscious. The appearance shocked all. Emaciated, hardly able to stand, their faces with large staring eyes were beyond pleading. Their stares were the stares of the desperate, bereft of hope.

Then there were the relatives, mainly parents but also wives, husbands, children, teenagers, adolescents, and young adults.

The role of the doctors of these patients was similarly a saga of desperation and helplessness, even hopelessness. There was little, if anything, they could do. In the absence of effective treatment, few in the medical profession chose to treat patients with diabetes.

Imagine then the excitement and desperate hope with which the news of a possible cure for the condition was greeted by the afflicted and their families when the discovery was described in a scientific journal by two Canadians in 1921 and, almost immediately, by the news media around the world.

The drama is captured by Bliss in the experience of one child. It was reported by the Boston physician Elliott Joslin in his first scientific paper on the subject of the effects of insulin on two children with diabetes.

An eight-year-old boy was carried into Joslin's office by his parents. He had been so hungry on his diet that he would burn his hands stealing food from a hot oven. "Dr. Joslin, do anything you want with Frederick, you can't make him any worse," his parents told Joslin.

After two months of insulin treatment, the mother wrote to Joslin that Frederick was feeling fine and wouldn't touch a particle of food other than his diet. He walked downtown every afternoon, the neighbourhood children staring in amazement at the little boy who had not been able to go out for the past two years.

> *"Nothing we can say based upon laboratory results can equal in importance statements of this character," Joslin and his associates concluded in the account of this case in their first paper on insulin. The same paper included the account of a little Finnish child who came into hospital, sank towards coma, was given insulin, and within 36 hours sat up in bed, played at the window, and threw a kiss to the doctor as he left her room.*
> Michael Bliss in *The Discovery of Insulin*.

The background to the discovery is one of the most dramatic and colourful chapters in the annals of the history of modern medicine.

Only when we look back at the times before the discovery of insulin does the magnitude of the change brought about by this discovery become clear.

A history of insulin cannot be separated from the history of diabetes.

Today, all round the world the number of adults afflicted with the condition has seen an alarming increase but this diabetes is different from that seen in young people and children. The commoner form of diabetes, also called Type II Diabetes or the rather cumbersome, NIDDM, Non-Insulin-Dependent Diabetes Mellitus, usually affects men and women over the age of 40 years. It is almost always accompanied by obesity.

Insulin saved and dramatically changed the lives of countless children and young people. In these patients there is a loss of the production of insulin because the cells in the body which make insulin have been destroyed by the body itself. The term autoimmune diabetes refers to this condition. At other times diabetes is seen after viral infections such as that recorded many years ago when an epidemic of mumps in parts of Scandinavia was followed by a significant rise in the number of patients developing diabetes. In many cases, however, diabetes develops for no apparent reason.

Diabetes in adults generally starts in middle-aged men and women who are frequently obese and have a comparatively inactive lifestyle. In such individuals, insulin is needed less frequently as these patients usually respond to dietary measures, and weight-loss. In addition, tablets can be taken to help further with keeping their blood sugar levels within an acceptable range.

In my work as a physician (internist) following graduation from the medical school at the University of Sydney in 1962 and then as a specialist in internal medicine and endocrinology (diabetes), I saw first-hand the remarkable effects of insulin on patients with diabetes. It is difficult to describe the transformation, within days of starting insulin, especially in the young. My experiences and observations were made 40 to 50 years after the discovery of insulin. Far more interesting and thought-provoking are the stories told by physicians who were treating patients with diabetes before the discovery of insulin.

For doctors and patients alike there is nothing quite as illuminating as reading the impressions and experiences of those who saw both sides of this story, namely the situation of patients and their carers before the discovery of insulin, then the drama at the time of the discovery followed by the remarkable transformations, as well as some disappointments, frustrations and challenges during the time that followed the discovery.

Two physicians who had this experience were Frederick Madison Allen (1879–1964) and Elliott Proctor Joslin (1869 –1962).

In 1969 my wife and I travelled with our two daughters to Boston where I worked at the Joslin Clinic as a Fellow in Diabetes and Internal Medicine for two years.

At the time I had not realised that Dr Joslin had worked till the last day of his life of nearly 93 years and had died only seven years before I started my fellowship. It was impossible to walk through the various buildings of the New England Deaconess Hospital, of which he was the first and Chief Physician, as well as the building housing the Joslin Clinic without sensing that the very structures of these institutions were imbued with the spirit of that remarkable man.

Joslin had treated thousands of men, women and children with diabetes in the 20 years before the discovery of insulin and even greater numbers over the 40 years afterwards. Highly respected throughout the English speaking world, Joslin was regarded by some as the greatest diabetologist of the 20th century.

Elliott Proctor Joslin (1869 –1962)

This book follows my study of the life of Dr Elliott Proctor Joslin (1869-1962), *Joslin A Pioneer in Diabetes Care* which was published in 2019 to mark the 150th anniversary of his birth. Joslin had started his medical practice following an internship at Massachusetts General Hospital in 1898 and had developed an early interest in diabetes. In 1916, several years before the discovery of insulin, he published the first textbook on diabetes in English. The breadth of his first-hand experience in treating diabetes before and after the introduction of insulin was described in lucid prose in his textbooks and instruction manuals each of which he produced in 10 editions and released at regular intervals over a period of some 40 years. The Boston physician and Harvard professor was generally regarded as being without peer in the treatment of diabetes in the United States and perhaps in the entire English-speaking world at that time.

There were other physicians who also had considerable experience and expertise in the treatment of diabetes before the discovery of insulin. The names of Frederick Madison Allen and Rollin Woodyatt immediately spring to mind. However these were men in the United States and not in Toronto where the discovery was made. Their contributions are also included in this book.

Joslin's excellent writings which can be found in his letters to the many researchers involved in the discovery of insulin paint a very clear picture of the condition before the discovery of insulin. His emotional tribute to the fathers of the early years like Pavy and Bouchardat in the preface of the third edition of his textbook includes descriptions of the milestones in the search for insulin culminating in its discovery in 1921.

The fact that Joslin was one of the earliest physicians to describe the effects of insulin in previously untreated patients provides an invaluable fund of knowledge and insight into the parlous state of those who suffered from diabetes in those early times. The discovery of insulin brought about the remarkable improvements of a magnitude that defied description. His comments and material from his books written for the public in his instruction manuals and for physicians in his textbook on diabetes are quoted as epigrams and also within the body of this work.

The physical and emotional states of individuals with diabetes before the discovery of insulin can be deduced from the transformation with the treatment with insulin as described in biblical terms by Joslin especially in his instruction manuals for patients.

Frederick Madison Allen (1879– 1964)

Whereas Joslin excelled in communicating with patients as well as physicians, an equally well known physician was Frederick Madison Allen who demonstrated his capacity for unrelenting effort at conducting animal experiments on literally thousands of animals to produce diabetes and then studied its effects. He also treated large numbers of patients in his hospital in New York. Allen pioneered the use of restricted diets as virtually the only method of keeping patients with diabetes alive but at the cost of making them extremely thin. The appearance of such patients and Allen's insistence on strict adherence to the diet made him unpopular and therefore not as widely respected as the charismatic Joslin. The two physicians were friends and each supported the other throughout his life. We will return to Dr Allen in the halcyon days of the summer of 1922.

There is much to be said for the use of chronology to trace the progress of a scientific mission, in this case the pursuit of the "internal secretion," thought to be the cause of diabetes before the discovery and identification of insulin.

The gifted physician and writer Siddhartha Mukherjee rightly suggests that transitions of scientific thought on a given subject are a useful way to present a narrative of scientific endeavour.

I have also traced chronologically the steps which lead to solving the riddle including some of the experiments which changed the thinking on the nature of insulin and brought about a transition in, or a progression to, the various concepts held on the nature of this fascinating protein. Scientific advances unlocked secrets which had for centuries mystified, even mocked the efforts of mere mortals including the most gifted.

My own habit when studying historic subjects has been to do so through the lives of those involved in such studies. Using this method I met remarkable men and women at different stages in the pursuit of insulin. The stories and scholastic efforts and accomplishments of the many physicians and researchers in the insulin story frequently reveal stories within stories.

My decision to tell the story of insulin in the centenary year of its discovery was because of my interest in the effects of insulin especially in young patients throughout my years in consultant practice.

Having seen first-hand how insulin changed the lives of patients suffering from diabetes as well as it's profound influence on the parents and other relatives caring for patients, I feel that celebrating the centenary of this remarkable "elixir of life" for millions is appropriate.

Except in the two books already mentioned, the dramatic changes in the treatment of diabetes with insulin have been written about only in medical journals but have received little attention in any comprehensive description of insulin since its discovery in 1921.

The treatment of diabetes achieved with changes in many insulin preparations as well as the methods of their delivery has resulted in dramatic improvements in the day-to-day management of those afflicted with the condition.

Advances through research particularly in molecular chemistry and genetics have culminated in the capacity for synthesising insulin without reliance on animal sources as had been the case for much of the first 100 years since its discovery in Toronto.

The story of what can be called "modern" insulin has its own cast of colourful characters and collection of fascinating stories and anecdotes.

The world-wide effects of Covid, rightly referred to as a pandemic, make it particularly important to appreciate that diabetes had reached epidemic proportions in much of the developed world more than fifty years ago and is now also affecting some of the third-world countries.

I hope that this book, in spite of its many shortcomings, may provide interesting reading not only for those who use insulin but also the wider community including social and political stakeholders especially since there is now an increased awareness of the pandemic of diabetes.

PART ONE
INSULIN PURSUED

DIABETES AN ANCIENT MALADY

It is thought-provoking that diabetes was known to man for several thousand years before the birth of Christ, its beginnings shrouded in the mists of antiquity dating back to the times of the pharaohs of Egypt.

The written history of diabetes begins in the second millennium. In the second century BC the Egyptians recorded their entire fund of knowledge in 42 secret books. Their medical knowledge was contained in the last six of these. However, the details remained hidden from history until the 19th century when Egyptologists began finding the Egyptian papyri which contained knowledge of medical matters. These were considered to be the oldest and most important medical papyri of ancient Egypt.

Yet it was only in 1874 through the work of German Egyptologist called George Moritz Ebers (1837–1898) that the early history of diabetes came to light.

The youngest of five children from a wealthy family which included bankers and merchants, George Ebers was born in Berlin. He was raised by his mother, his father having died shortly after Ebers's birth. He studied at Gottingen where, in addition to jurisprudence, oriental languages and archaeology, he had devoted a good deal of time to a special study of the Egyptian language and history. In 1870 he was appointed Professor in these subjects.

In the winter of 1873–1874 during a visit to Luxor (Thebes), Ebers had discovered the Egyptian papyri and in 1875 he bought what later came to be known as the Ebers papyrus. These, together with the Edwin Smith Papyrus (circa 1600 BCE) and the Ibis papyrus (circa 1550 BCE) are regarded as the oldest preserved medical documents anywhere.

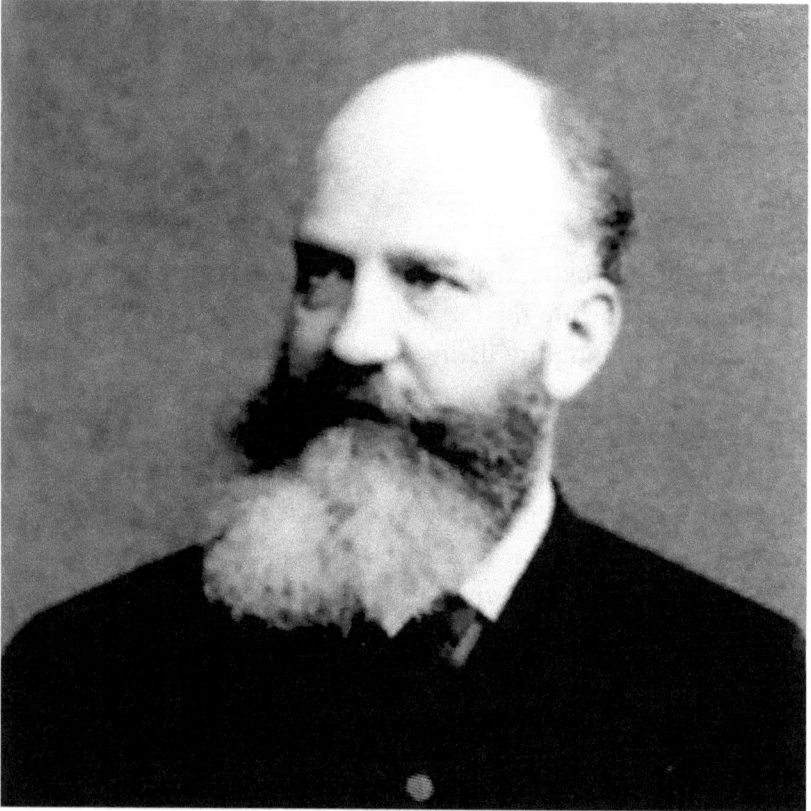

Georg Ebers German professor discovered Egyptian papyrus.

In 1875 George Ebers published the first of what are frequently referred to collectively as the Ebers Papyrus. It is said to be a 110 page scroll, 20 meters long and is considered to be amongst the oldest preserved medical documents. Ebers published the papyrus as a facsimile adding English letters and vocabulary. He also provided an introduction.

The contents of this document included descriptions of life in general. The breadth of knowledge in those ancient times was breathtaking to say the least. The papyri as they came to be known – published as a facsimile – noted 700 different substances and medical recipes including incantations and concoctions.

Not only was diabetes known to the ancients but they actually described the treatment for it.

The treatment of diabetes recommended in this document was a mixture including elderberry, asit plant fibres, milk, beer-swill, cucumber flowers and green dates. The exact nature of the plant called acit remains obscure.

Emhotep, said to be Chancellor and Doctor of the king of Egypt, the Pharaoh Djoser around 27th century BCE, is credited with, among other attributes, knowledge of medical conditions and treatment.

According to William Osler, regarded by many as the father of modern medicine and the greatest physician of the 20th century, Emhotep was "the first figure of a physician to stand out clearly from the mesh of antiquity."

Pertinent to this account of diabetes is the description by Emhotep of excessive passage of urine (polyuria) which would arguably place the initial description of diabetes as far back as 2650 BC.

Another Egyptian physician, Hesy-Ra – in 1550 2BC documented frequent urination as a symptom of a mysterious disease that also caused emaciation. Physicians of the time also noted that ants seemed to gather around the urine of people who had this disease.

What should be noted is the gap of nearly 3000 years between the period of Egyptian medicine and the Greek or Roman period mentioned next.

Claudius Galenus, (125–199 A.D.), the renowned Roman physician used the term "diarrhoea urinosa."

Today diabetes, the term which is used in English-speaking countries is said to be a transliteration of a Greek word which means "passing through" or "siphon".

Aretaeus of Cappadocia (about 150 A.D.) is credited with a detailed description of diabetes and is quoted in the 13th edition of Joslin's Diabetes Mellitus (editors C. Ronald Kahn and Gordon C. Weir published by Lea Febiger, 1994.)

Diabetes is a remarkable disorder, and not one very common to man. It consists of a moist and cold wasting of the flesh and limbs into urine, from a cause similar to that of dropsy; the secretion passes in the usual way, by the kidneys and bladder. The patients never cease making water, but the discharge is as incessant as a sluice let off. This disease is chronic in character, and is slowly enough gendered, though the patient does not survive long when it is completely established for the marasmus produced is rapid and death is speedy.

The Indian physician Sushruta and the surgeon Charaka (400–500 AD) described diabetes as *madhumeha* which literally translated means "honey urine."

The next star on the horizon of the history of diabetes was a remarkable Persian polymath called Avicenna (980–1037), also known as Ibn Sina. Respected and admired as a thinker and writer, Avicenna, regarded by some as the father of early modern medicine, as well as one of the most knowledgeable astronomers, physicians and thinkers of that period which was often called the golden age of Islam. He was born in Afshona, Uzbekistan in August 980 A.D. and died on June 22, 1037 in Iran.

Avicenna described excessive appetite and, remarkably, one of the complications of diabetes, gangrene. That this remains one of the most feared complications of diabetes even today emphasises the long history of the frustrations and helplessness experienced by the afflicted and those charged with the management of the complications of diabetes.

Little wonder that one of the modern American diabetologists, Arthur Colwell (1924-2018), referred to the pre-insulin years as the "frustration era."

Why then did it take thousands of years to address the problem of treating diabetes?

Put simply, because even though the main effect of diabetes, namely the excessive passage of urine, was described all those thousands of years ago, the actual nature of the underlying condition was not known.

A prevailing view of illness in ancient times was the belief that any illness was a manifestation of divine will, usually a punishment for some perceived wrongdoing on the part of those afflicted. In some societies even today such convictions hold sway resulting in the segregation that those who happen to be affected by conditions ranging from leprosy and tuberculosis to, in recent times, AIDS.

Prejudice towards those suffering from diabetes persists in many communities to this day.

Yet the nature of diabetes has only been elucidated in the last 100 years. The reason lies in the remarkable change in the thinking on the nature of illness as described in the writings of scholars in several European medical schools. Before then, illness was thought to result from various ill-defined forces of nature which were peculiar to human beings. The chief proponent of this was Aristotle but prominent physicians including Galen and Paracelsus also shared this view.

Other beliefs which held sway maintained that illness was visited upon humans by the will of the gods or that they were natural phenomena such as evil influences which were best avoided rather than studied. Superstitions and supernatural forces playing a role also had their followers in many human societies.

The gods were not to be questioned.

This so-called vitalistic nature of illness began to be questioned in the 18th and more so in the 19th century. However, prominent medical pioneers including Louis Pasteur (1822–1895) are said to have performed experiments which suggested that he may have supported vitalism.

SEARCHING FOR THE SOURCE, THE "SEAT" OF DIABETES

The Strange Case of an Oxford Professor who tasted urine.

Thomas Willis (1621–1675), had introduced the term diabetes mellitus in 1674. Willis was a professor of natural philosophy at Oxford and tasted the urine of diabetic patients which he found to be sweet. As already stated this characteristic of urine from diabetic patients had been described several hundred years earlier.

Almost exactly 100 years later in 1776 Matthew Dobson of Manchester in England demonstrated that diabetic urine actually contained sugar. Evaporation through boiling produced crystals which were brown in colour and tasted sweet. Dobson referred to these as "brown sugar". Dobson's findings led to questions on the possible organs of the body which produced this brown sugar. At first the kidneys were believed to be the seat of the disease because the diabetic had to pass urine frequently. Later it was realised that the condition also made the patients pass copious amounts of urine over a 24 hour period.

The sweetness of urine was likened to honey in the writings of the early Arabian and other Eastern scholars. There were further questions when the sweetness was shown to be due to sugar by the Englishman John Rollo who at that time was the Surgeon-General of the Royal Artillery.

Rollo was an interesting character with a background in colonial administration. He had spent a good deal of time in the West Indies where cultivation of sugarcane was an important industry dependent on slave-labour from Africa and later, indentured workers from India.

However Rollo is credited with being the first to use Dobson's method for measuring urinary glucose in quantitative metabolic studies of diabetes.

Furthermore he devised the first rational approach to the dietary treatment of diabetes and changed the thinking on the "seat" of diabetes from the kidneys to the gut.

In 1797 Rollo wrote a book on diabetes,

"An account of two cases of diabetes mellitus with remarks as they arose during the progress of the cure. To which are added a general view of the nature of the disease and its appropriate treatment."

The book was re-published some years later. However, apart from confirming that the sweetness of diabetic urine was due to sugar, the book contributed little else to the understanding of the condition at that time. Rollo had used Dobson's method of testing for the presence of glucose in urine of his diabetic patients.

In 1788 Cawley reported in detail the post-mortem findings in a single case when he described – without comment – a shrivelled pancreas which also contains stones. The authors in the Joslin textbook (13th edition) observed that this may have been the first published reference to the pancreas in relation to human diabetes but noted that no deductions were drawn as to its possible role in the cause of diabetes.

It was Rollo's continuing interest in the presence of sugar in the urine that resulted in an important change in the thinking of the doctors interested in the disorder at that time. To further study the loss of sugar in the urine discovered by Dobson, he engaged in one of the first metabolic studies on diabetes. In order to record the type and amount of food being consumed by one of his patients, a Captain Meredith described by Rollo as "a corpulent man with adult onset diabetes with severe bladder coryza," Rollo carried out daily weight recordings of the amount and kinds of food eaten, then weighing the sugar cake obtained by boiling and evaporating the urine each day.

The critical effect of these studies was to shift the thinking on the cause of diabetes from the kidney to the gut. Rollo proposed that the loss of sugar in the urine was simply a reflection of overproduction of sugar from vegetable matter in the stomach. He said that the "morbid" organ of diabetes was therefore not the kidney but the "stomach."

This was possibly the first step taken on the path of the treatment of diabetes with a reduction in carbohydrate (starch) intake and one which remained the mainstay of treatment until the discovery of insulin more than 100 years later.

But there is more to the insulin story.

Rollo had assumed that hyperglycaemia existed in diabetes but early attempts to measure "sugar" in the blood failed because of the assumption that sugar in the food was the same as table sugar.

In 1815 Chevruil showed that blood sugar behaved chemically as "grape" sugar or glucose. Further developments in methodology showed that the "reducing substance" in serum and urine was indeed glucose.

These findings confirmed Rollo's earlier predictions that in diabetes it is an increase in the level of glucose in the blood which leads to the loss of glucose in the urine. Therefore the underlying abnormality in diabetes must lie somewhere other than in the kidneys.

Getting closer to the "seat" of the problem

French Connections.

Many physicians in Europe and England especially Germany and France suspected the role of the pancreas in causing diabetes. They knew of the presence of diabetes in patients with post-mortem findings of abnormalities in this organ. Frequently the pancreas was scarred and shrunken. At other times, it was filled with numerous tiny stones (calculi). A major obstacle to accepting the pancreas as the seat of the abnormality causing diabetes arose from the fact that in the vast majority of cases the pancreas appeared completely normal in post-mortem examination of diabetic patients. It is important to appreciate that even the role of the pancreas in digestion was only just being accepted by medical practitioners of that era.

Therefore the existence of the abnormalities in the organ described above in the post-mortem examination of diabetics was considered to be a chance finding and of no significance as far as the cause of diabetes was concerned.

An important reason for dismissing the "pancreatic theory" was the stand taken by Claude Bernard, a highly respected scientist throughout Europe and the English – speaking world. To test the role of the pancreas as a cause of diabetes, Bernard carried out experiments in dogs. By tying off or injecting paraffin in the pancreatic duct he blocked, the production of pancreatic juice by the organ. This led to pronounced shrinking (atrophy) of the pancreas leaving only tiny shrivelled remnants which Bernard considered insignificant. Yet the experimental animals showed no signs of diabetes. His results were published in a French medical journal in 1850. Bernard was not the only scientist to have used this information to cast serious doubt on the "pancreatic theory" as a cause of diabetes.

Krall, Levine, and Barnett, the authors of the chapter on the history of diabetes in *Joslin's Diabetes Mellitus* (13th edition), consider Claude Bernard's opinions an important reason for the pancreas not being considered of any importance as a cause of diabetes for a period of up to 50 years (1830–1880).

Therefore it is pertinent to look at Bernard's background and work which led to the high regard in which he was, and continues to be, held in the medical and scientific world.

Claude Bernard, a Peerless Scientist

Claude Bernard (1813–1878) was a highly respected scientist and physician. Born in a small village called Saint-Julien near Villefranche-sur-Saone, Bernard went to college in Lyon but left to become an assistant in a chemist shop. Initially his interest was in drama which took him to Paris where a music critic persuaded him to go to medical school. He became an Intern at the Hotel-Dieu de Paris where the highly respected but controversial physiologist Francois Magendie was the professor. Bernard, aware and conscious of his Chief's experience and knowledge of physiology, discussed with him the speculations and autopsy findings and their relevance to the possible role of the pancreas in causing diabetes.

Magendie, who was no stranger to controversy, even criticism (for live dissections of animals at public lectures on physiology), gently pointed out to his enthusiastic younger colleague that the role of the pancreas being a cause of diabetes in light of Bernard's "presentation" was at best a hypothesis. He urged the young investigator to devise an experiment to test this hypothesis.

The young man proceeded to do just that. Using dogs for this purpose Bernard tied off the ducts within the pancreas – the pancreatic duct usually has one main channel but often also has several smaller ones – which normally carry the pancreatic juice out of the gland into the gut to break down food materials for digestion. Bernard's experiment revealed that most of the pancreas was destroyed and all that remained was a collection of filaments or threads which Bernard assumed had no significance. He confidently concluded that his experiment had succeeded in causing total destruction (atrophy) of the pancreas. Furthermore he found that the dogs did not develop diabetes. Therefore he felt confident that he could dismiss pancreas is being the seat of diabetes.

The results of these experiments together with the impeccable reputation of Magendie in physiology halted further investigation of the pancreas for its role in diabetes. Other organs including the brain were then pursued by Bernard.

After a period as deputy professor, Bernard succeeded Magendie, becoming a full professor in 1855. His brilliance as a researcher surpassed Magendie.

Bernard Cohen of Harvard University called Claude Bernard "one of the greatest of all men of science."

In spite of Bernard's views, not all physicians were totally persuaded of the innocence of the pancreas. Abnormalities in the organ continued to be seen in patients with diabetes. Ironically the two clinicians most often quoted as considering that the pancreas was the organ responsible for diabetes were, like Bernard, Frenchman. They were not as quick as some to dismiss the post-mortem findings of scarred and shrivelled pancreases. Etienne Lancereaux (1829–1910) had observed the difference between the severe form of diabetes in thin patients and the less severe form, which he called "diabetes of the fat".

Lancereaux's work had been observed and noted by his assistant, a Romanian scholar called Nicolas Constantin Paulescu (1869–1931). Neither could have known at the time the part which the young man was going to play in the history of the discovery of insulin as will be seen later in the story.

An even more prominent French physician was Apollinaire Bouchardat, referred to by Elliott Joslin as "the Prince of Physicians." Ironically, Bouchardat was also working at the Hotel-Dieu, the hospital where Bernard had worked and from where his findings on the pancreas were published in 1850.

He had carried out long-term studies on patients with diabetes and had in 1875 written one of the earliest textbooks on the subject, *De la Glycosuria ou Diabete Sucre*.

Bouchardat had used Rollo's recommendations for diet for diabetics.

Two other important contributions to the treatment of diabetics were originally made by Bouchardat. Firstly, he added exercise to the treatment regime of adult (type two) diabetics because he had observed that hard work reduced the amount of sugar lost in the urine. Secondly he distinguished two different types of diabetes, namely the severe (Type one) affecting the young and (Type two) in the obese adults.

The two French physicians suggested that the severe diabetes of the young was from pancreatic damage and was more resistant to dietary treatment then the adult form which benefited from a diet causing weight loss.

Bouchardat worked in the renowned hospital, which is operational to this day, to the end of his life. He died in poverty and was buried in the Pere Lachaise cemetery in Paris. The Boston physician and diabetes specialist Elliott Joslin on his many trips to Paris never left the city without visiting Bouchardat's grave.

DEATH OF A MEDICAL LUMINARY BY GUILLOTINE

Antoine-Laurent Lavoisier (1743-1794)

Lavoisier was born to a wealthy family of French nobility and the son of a prominent lawyer. His grounding in science was from his interest in meteorological observation under the tutelage of Nicholas Louis de Lacaille, a distinguished mathematician and observational astronomer. These interests continued even though Lavoisier studied and received a law degree and was admitted to the bar.

He had also studied chemistry and his work in that field made basic contributions to the understanding of human physiology and biochemistry relating to food and nutrition. His work established the value of the respiratory quotient and measurement of oxygen consumption at rest, following exercise, and importantly, food ingestion and digestion.

During the French Revolution, because of his association with a government agency which collected tax on behalf of the King, Lavoisier was arrested along with all the other employees of that agency. Officially the charge was that they had all defrauded the state of money. They were also charged with adding water to tobacco before selling the product. Lavoisier drafted the defence but the court condemned all the accused and seized their goods. The judge declared that "the republic needs neither scholars nor chemists."

Lavoisier was guillotined on May 8, 1794 aged 50. He was pardoned one year later–one year too late.

Lavoisier's importance to science can be gauged from the lamentation of a colleague:

"It took them only an instant to cut off his head, and 100 years might not suffice to reproduce his like."

An Earlier Epidemic and a Young Victim

"Your young men will see visions."

Joel, an Israeli prophet.

PAUL LANGERHANS

Paul Langerhans was born into a family of physicians. He was the son of a respected doctor, Paul Augustus Langerhans who practised in Berlin where young Paul was born in 1847.

In 1865 at the age of 18, he graduated from high school and went to the university in the historic town of Jena, an ancient city which is described in documents dating back to the ninth century. Today it is famous for its collection of Zeiss microscopes and spectacles.

Towards the end of his course Langerhans transferred to the University of Berlin where the teaching faculty included the distinguished medical scholar Rudolph Virchow (1821–1902).

Virchow impressed on his students the importance of using the microscope in investigating disease.

"Think microscopically," he urged.

In 1869, using light microscopy, Langerhans described the cells of the pancreas, a comma-shaped organ lying behind the stomach and concerned mainly with breaking down (digestion) of food particles. Although many of the varieties of cells he described were known at the time, his description also contained a clear account of one type of cell which had not been noticed previously. These were seen as small collections (clusters) scattered throughout the pancreas. They looked distinctly different from the others.

Langerhans did not attempt to claim any particular function for these cells. He expressed no opinion on what purpose they served.

His findings were contained in his thesis presented in 1869 with the title "Contributions to the Microscopic Anatomy of the Pancreas."

At the time of this discovery Langerhans was 22 years old.

He remained with Virchow for another year but was enlisted to serve in the Franco-Prussian war in 1870. On his return he served as a professor of pathology in Freiburg. A few years after his war service Langerhans developed tuberculosis in his kidneys. Even though he responded to treatment at first he never regained his strength and died in 1888 at the age of 41.

It is a fact of history that scant attention was paid to the work a medical student had carried out in 1869 until many years later.

OSKAR MINKOWSKI (1858–1931)

The horse wins the race, the jockey takes the cup.

Edgar Degas.

Minkowski was born in the riverside town of Alexoten in Russia, now called Alexotas in Lithuania, across the river from today's Kaunas. He came from a family which carried impeccable academic and social credentials. His older brother Max was a prosperous businessman and had served as the French Consul in Konigsberg. His younger brother Herman was a world renowned mathematician – one of his students was Albert Einstein.

Oskar Minkowski himself had received an excellent education, having attended the famous Alstadter gymnasium in Konigsberg and later, the medical faculty of the University of Freiburg and Konigsberg, the latter known for the philosopher Emanuel Kant being on its teaching faculty.

Minkowski pursued an illustrious career not only as an academic and researcher but also as a highly respected practising physician with expertise in diabetes and internal medicine. Amongst the better known of his patients was the Russian leader Vladimir Ilyich Lenin.

Oskar Minkowski died in 1931 at the age of 73 years.

His was the most important discovery to that point in time because it settled the question of the organ involved. As related above, attention had shifted from the kidneys because of the sweet urine, to the stomach because of the alterations in the composition of the urine depending on the food eaten. After this the pancreas was suspected and then dismissed as the organ responsible.

Minkowski's Surgical Skill and Medical Intuition.

In April 1889, Minkowski went to the Biochemical Institute to read some recent publications and met von Mering who in the course of conversation said, "healthy people must metabolise lipids and if the pancreas doesn't work correctly, we have to give metabolised lipids to them."

"Did you prove this in an experiment?" asked Minkowski.

This was followed by a discussion on how to do the experiment and finally, Minkowski mentioned that the question could be studied in a dog.

Minkowski did not know that Claude Bernard had stated that no animal survived a total pancreatectomy and perhaps over-estimating his capability as a surgeon famously declared,

"There are no impossible operations. Give me a dog. I will take out his pancreas today." von Mering agreed to let Minkowski proceed.

The same day Minkowski performed a total pancreatectomy in a dog in Naunyn's laboratory with the assistance of von Mering.

The animal survived and seemed to be doing well in the beginning but within twenty four hours started to urinate more and more frequently in the laboratory. Minkowski reprimanded the laboratory assistant for not walking the dog frequently enough but the young man replied, "I do walk him frequently but this animal's funny. As soon as it returns, it urinates again even immediately after having done it outside."

This observation led Minkowski to examine the urine of the dog. The rest, as they say, is history.

The presence of glucose in the urine confirmed that the pancreas was the seat of the problem causing diabetes and assured

Minkowski a pride of place in medical history. He is often referred to as the "father of diabetes".

Minkowski was 31 years old when he made this critical observation. It must also be mentioned that Josef von Mering was only 40.

Minkowski never forgot what von Mering had done for him, and, from the point of view of medical history, for the seminal discovery attributed to the young investigator. In the scientific publications of the experiment Minkowski placed his colleague's name before his own out of respect not only because von Mering was older but also because he had supported, if not encouraged, the enthusiastic young man to undertake the surgery. It was von Mering who had provided the dog.

Minkowski pursued a distinguished medical career and was feted throughout the world. He was nominated for the Nobel Prize at least six times but never won it.

History has been less considerate of von Mering's contribution. The selfless, tall nobleman of striking bearing who was also admired as a swordsman had been largely forgotten in the Insulin story.

But fate did not forget him.

One of the latest drugs, Sglt 2 inhibitors, introduced in the treatment of diabetes draws on experimental work originally carried out by von Mering.

Gustave Edouard Laguesse. (1861-1927.)

Almost exactly 20 years after the description by Langerhans of the clusters of cells in the pancreas, Laguesse while studying the pancreas of fish made an invaluable contribution.

Laguesse was born in Dijon, the capital of Burgundy, an area known for its mustard farms and beautiful vineyards. In 1889, when he was 28 years old, he suggested that the clusters of cells described by Langerhans discharged their product directly into the blood. He predicted that these clusters of cells produced insulin and gave them the name the "islets of Langerhans" which remains the term used for them to this day.

Laguesse is not often mentioned in the story of diabetes but his critical contribution did not go unnoticed by the French scientific community. One of their leaders commented that "Laguesse deduced from his observations something which has made his name worthy of commemoration forever by biologists and physicians namely, the concept of the endocrine role of the Islets of Langerhans the development of which led to the practical discovery of insulin as it appears from the very name given to this physiological medicament. Of course, Langerhans had noticed them but only as a navigator who notes in his logbook an archipelago which happens to live within the range of his outlook at sea. Laguesse was the Explorer who passed on the same route, halted at these "terra Incogniti", went ashore, mapped and surveyed them so thoroughly that it was possible for later scholars to search them for resources for a new therapeutic agent."

PART TWO

INSULIN DISCOVERED

TORONTO WHERE IT ALL BEGAN

"Black-sheep sons and ne'er-do-wells"

The English settlers in Canada date their arrival in the colony from the early 1600s. Coopers Cove (now Cupid) was established by Royal Charter granted by James 1st to Bristol merchant John Gray in 1610. It was the first colony established by Royal assent in Canada and second only to Jamestown in Virginia for which the Royal Charter had been granted in 1607.

In addition to commercial advantages which in Newfoundland was mainly from fishing, the distant colonies also served as convenient settlements to which inconvenient relatives were transported and removed from the public eye at home in England and Ireland. One such story was of Tom, the unfortunate 19-year-old son of prominent English merchant entrepreneur Sir Percival Willoughby (1560–1643). Regarded as the black sheep of the family, the hapless young man was herded onto the second lot of colonists bound for Canada in 1612 and removed from the public eye or perhaps more importantly, the whispers and gossips in the village, and was never heard of again. The admonition of the local magistrate who had convicted the young man has been immortalised in inscriptions and is quoted frequently by Canadian historians.

"Thomas Willoughby, thou art a ne'er do well,
Get thee to Cupers Cove and reform thyself."

Thomas Willoughby's father, Sir Percival Willoughby continued to maintain a lofty presence amongst the wealthy in Nottinghamshire. (That is until his debtors caught up with him in his later years but that is a story for another day).

The city of Toronto, situated on Lake Ontario is a vibrant city with prominent commercial, industrial and cultural activities as befits the capital of the Province of Ontario.

It has a rich history, tracing its early inhabitants to the Ice Age. But until 1922, in the scientific and medical world, Toronto was not in the league of the medical and research centres of Europe and England. Nor could it boast of generations of illustrious medical teachers, researchers and scientists. All this changed in 1921 because of insulin.

THE SUMMER OF 1921

"We all have our feelings and prejudices. Even with the most careful adherence to the scientific method, it's difficult to see the world as it truly is. One has to be systematic, and observant of details. This takes a certain amount of bloody – mindedness and grit."
Scientia Professor Michelle Simmons,
FRS, AO, UNSW Science.
Winner of 2021 Bakerian Medal and Lecture.

"Be not afraid of greatness. Some are born great, some achieve greatness, and some have greatness thrust upon them."
William Shakespeare: Twelfth Night. Act 2, Scene 5

"To be yourself in a world that is constantly trying to make you something else is the greatest accomplishment."
Ralph Waldo Emerson.

FREDERICK "FRED" GRANT BANTING, A YOUNG MAN IN A HURRY

The summer of 1921 marked the beginning of Banting's search for "the elusive substance" which when deficient, caused diabetes but when present, prevented it. As already mentioned, two European scientists, Josef von Mering and Oskar Minkowski some 30 years earlier had dramatically demonstrated that the pancreas was the "seat" of diabetes.

It is of interest to relate the background especially the knowledge and experience of the main participants in the insulin story. They were Frederick Banting, Charles Best, Bertram Collip and James Macleod.

Controversies surrounding the discovery do not include any comparisons between the roles played by the man most closely associated with Banting namely, Charles Herbert Best. That Banting was the senior investigator and Best his assistant is one of the few points not in contention.

Best was a 4th-year student in the Physiology and Biochemistry course at the University of Toronto when he joined Banting during his (Best's) summer break. Students in this course frequently worked as demonstrators and research assistants to pick up extra pocket money. In the normal course of events these students went on to do a Masters of Arts degree which for Best would have been directed by the Head of the department, Professor John Macleod.

Frederick Grant Banting (1891–1941) initiated the research which culminated in the discovery of insulin. Banting had no delusions about his limitations as far as diabetes was concerned. When discussing this aspect of his background in 1940, many years after the discovery of insulin (1940). He said,

"I remember seeing one patient only on the wards of the Toronto General Hospital. There was no such thing as a diabetic ward in my surgical experience...

I did not even know that my friend and classmate Joe Gilchrist had diabetes until I had been mostly working on the problem for many months."

Fred Banting was born on November 14, 1891 in Alliston, the fifth son and the youngest of six in his family. Alliston at that time was a small town with a small population – even today its inhabitants number less than 20,000. His parents, Margaret Grant and William Thompson Banting had moved to Canada from Ireland. They were devout Methodists and hard-working farmers who observed the basic tenets of their faith including abstinence from alcohol. Fred had grown-up on the farm and attended local schools. His parents encouraged him to continue his education beyond the level of primary school. In 1910 Banting enrolled in an Arts course at Victoria College in the University of Toronto. However he was not able to pass all his subjects and had to repeat first year. During this year he learned that he could enter the faculty of medicine and promptly dropped out of the Arts course. Clearly he did not wish to follow the hope of his parents that he would enter the ministry. The University of Toronto was considered the best in that part of the country.

The transition from the small town of his birth to Canada's second largest city was an eye-opener for the young farm boy. He enrolled in the faculty of medicine in the autumn of 1912. Banting's grades in medical school were average and he certainly did not stand out academically. This was a period of World War I and the five–year program in medicine had been radically condensed. In December 1916, Banting graduated with a Bachelor's degree.

He did not consider himself to be particularly well trained and harboured serious doubts about his ability to engage in medical practice. The teaching hospital attached to the medical school, the recently rebuilt and very modern Toronto General Hospital occupied pride of place in the city and, as will be seen later in this account, in the scientific world. Aspects of medical research were introduced early to the aspiring doctor because of the emphasis on investigations especially in physiology. His chief character trait seems to have been a dogged determination to stick to whatever tasks he was assigned. Socially awkward, he was said to have "two Methodist feet" when it came to dancing. Although only an average student Banting was better at sport preferring athletics to studies. Most of his spare time was spent with Edith Roach, the daughter of the minister of the Methodist church in Banting's hometown of Alliston.

The 1914 –1918 war shortened his medical course. In later years he often commented that he had "a very deficient medical training," often claiming that he had only five pages of notes for the entire final year. Physically imposing – he was 6 foot tall and good looking – Banting had served in the Canadian Medical Army Corps for two years and had then gone to England in 1917. Prior to leaving for military duties he had become engaged to Edith Roach.

He had seen action as a battalion medical officer on the front and during one engagement was seriously wounded by a shrapnel in the arm. He had continued to engage the enemy even when asked to withdraw and was later awarded the Military Cross for courage under fire. The action had occurred during the engagement at Cambria.

Banting convalesced in Britain before returning to Toronto in March 1919. Significant from the point of view of his later research is that much of Banting's surgical experience came from treating wounds during his war service in the summer of 1918.

It must be noted however that while in England he had devoted his free time to studying and had obtained the membership to the Royal College of Surgeons. He was also developing an interest in research the details of which are scant. There was certainly no mention of any interest in diabetes at that time.

In 1920 Banting, aged 29 was a World War I veteran and a well trained doctor. He was no longer the temperate Methodist of his youth but rather a veteran with what Bliss called "the veterans' usual minor vices – drinking, swearing, and heavy smoking."

After the war Banting rejoined Clarence Starr, the much admired Chief Surgeon at the Hospital for Sick Children in Toronto. He did a residency in paediatric orthopaedic surgery but most of his surgical experience had been gained during his time as a surgeon on the front during his active war service in France during the First World War.

Much to his disappointment, Banting was not invited back to The Hospital for Sick Children upon completion of his residency.

So in 1918 Frederick Banting, who was then 28 years old, had no alternative but to go into general practice. He borrowed money from his father to buy a modest cottage in London, Ontario and opened his office on July 1, 1920. London had been his choice because his fiancé Edith Roach was a teacher in a high school near there.

Unfortunately things didn't go well for Fred as he failed to attract enough patients to pay off a recently bought second-hand car, let alone make much of an impression on the money owed on the house.

To make ends meet he decided to accept a part-time position as a demonstrator in surgery at Western University in London where he started in October 1920. He was paid two dollars an hour.

As happens in the lives of many men and women when they are at their lowest ebb, a fortuitous acquaintance can sometimes lead to long-term consequences. Banting's work at Western University led to an acquaintance with F.W. Miller, a medical graduate and a highly respected physiologist who was later (in 1914) appointed as the first full Professor of Physiology at Western University. Miller, a devoted and brilliant academic, had a gift for teaching and kindling in his students an interest in human and animal experimentation.

It was with Miller that Banting first experienced the excitement of experimental physiology in particular and investigative medicine in general. Miller encouraged his students to conduct animal experiments in order to gain an insight into human physiology. At the time Miller was conducting animal experiments on stimulation of various parts of the brain. Indeed Banting's participation with Miller resulted in a scientific publication.

Banting's first contribution to medical literature was in the prestigious journal, Brain: Volume 45, issue 1, June 1, 1922. The article, Observations On Cerebellar Stimulations listed as its authors F.O. Miller, MA, MB, and F.G. Banting MC, MB.[*]

It is important to emphasise this early introduction to medical research in order to put in perspective the general view that Banting's work on insulin had a background entirely devoid of any exposure to, or experience in, medical research. No one including Banting himself could have foreseen what lay in his future in the field of investigative medicine.

Certainly the farm boy did not realise that this introduction to medical research was a portent of things to come. The influence of Frederick Miller on Banting and therefore in the insulin story has not been given a place of any great significance. Yet it was Miller to whom Banting had turned initially to discuss his ideas when searching for the elusive internal secretion of the pancreas and it was Miller who had told him whom to consult for guidance. We will return to this critical and central issue in the insulin story shortly.

A student was assigned by Professor Macleod to help Banting. That student, as mentioned earlier, was 21-year-old Charles Best.

---

[*] This piece of information was brought to my attention by my friend and fellow-bibliophile Milton Roxanas, through another member of the Osler Club, Professor Rolando del Maestro.

CHARLES HERBERT BEST (1899 –1978)

Best was the son of Luella Fisher Best and Herbert Heustess Best, a doctor who ran a one-man general practice in West Pembroke, Maine. They were originally from Nova Scotia and had always regarded themselves as Canadian.

In 1915 Best graduated from high school and moved to Toronto.

In 1918 he joined the Canadian army and served in the 70th Battery of the Horse Artillery attaining the rank of Sergeant before serving overseas in Wales with the Second Canadian Tank Battalion. In 1919 he returned to Toronto to complete his undergraduate degree in physiology and biochemistry. The professor and head of the department was James Macleod.

In July 1920 Best became engaged to Margaret Hooper Mahon, the function taking place at the farm of his friend and classmate E. Clark Noble. Best and Noble were working as research assistants under the supervision of James Macleod in the spring of 1921.

After graduation in 1921 Best, at the suggestion of his professor obtained a holiday job assisting Frederick Banting whom Macleod had given a small room in which to pursue his (Banting's) idea of seeking the internal secretion of the pancreas which Banting believed might provide a solution for the cause of diabetes.

This time with Banting would prove to be life changing for Best.

Best's entry into the pursuit of the elusive internal secretion is dealt with only briefly in Bliss's book including a story about his appointment being decided by the toss of a coin which at best can be viewed as a journalistic whim and at worst, trivialisation of Best's association with the project.

The role played by Best in the early stages of assessing the efficacy or even the suitability of the extract becomes clearer when his academic credentials are viewed.

At the time when Macleod had arranged for Charles Best to assist Banting in April 1921, Best had completed an honours degree in physiology and biochemistry. Initially the appointment was only for around six weeks – mid May to the end of June – at which time Best was required to attend compulsory army training, "militia camp" for 10 days.

In the fourth and final year of the course Best had undertaken a research project involving the production of diabetes by stimulating a part of the brain of a turtle. This was based on experiments conducted by Claude Bernard in the latter part of the previous century. Apart from being familiar with at least some of the literature on experimental aspects of diabetes, another feature of Best's practical training was in laboratory methods for estimating the amount of sugar (glucose) in small quantities of blood. As will be seen later, this technique which required only a very small volume of blood to be collected from the experimental subject was to play an important practical role in the insulin story.

Lastly, fourth-year students were also given weekly lectures, lasting two hours, by Macleod, on "The History and Present Knowledge of the Use of Sugars in the Body." These lectures had made Best aware of some of the work being done by American researchers including Woodyatt and Allen as well as Europeans including Hans Christian Hagedorn and earlier workers like August Krogh. Some of these men will figure prominently later in more than one part of this story.

However any evaluation of Best's contribution to Banting's project would need to be mindful of the fact that Charles Best was still a student and his laboratory experience was limited to exercises which were part of the curriculum of his university course. There is no record of any original scientific work being undertaken by him during his years as a student.

Of particular relevance in the context of the experiments planned by Banting are the opinions on "Sugar metabolism" expressed by Macleod in a book he had written. *Physiology and Biochemistry in Modern Medicine* was published in 1918. It was used as a textbook by his students.

A paragraph from this book is revealing. Firstly, Macleod did not believe that "any one enzyme or hormone" was essential in "sugar metabolism."

The paragraph reads:

"The removal of some hormone necessary for proper sugar metabolism is, however, by no means the only way by which the results can be explained, for we can assume that the pancreas owes its influence over sugar metabolism to some change occurring in the composition of the blood as it circulates through the gland – a change which is dependent on the integrity of the gland and not on any one enzyme or hormone which it produces."

The obvious question in this regard is why Macleod didn't tell Banting about this. Neither for that matter did Best who had attended lectures by Macleod on this subject and was familiar with the book referred to above. One could speculate that the fresh-faced young graduate, some 10 years younger than Banting, regarded this time with the older man as simply a job in his summer holidays to supplement his meagre income at the time. Presumably the payment was to be made by Banting as Macleod had made it clear to Best that the department did not have sufficient funds to pay him.

Thus it is clear that Best's knowledge on insulin was limited to the information provided by Macleod's lectures on the history of diabetes as well as the physiology and biochemistry of carbohydrates.

Still, given Banting's shortened medical course because of the 1914–1918 war, Charles Best's limited laboratory experience in carrying out some of the experimental procedures which were needed in the research being planned by the 30-year-old surgeon actually turned out to be of considerable help to Banting.

On the other hand, when it came to application of the knowledge which had been imparted to Best in his student days there is little evidence of any significant contribution by way of information or methodology when he began his time with Banting in May 1921.

For Best this time with Banting would proved to be life-changing

JOHN JAMES RICKARD MACLEOD (1876-1935)

Much has been written about James Macleod, especially on his sharing the Nobel Prize with Banting. It is therefore pertinent to describe the scholastic achievements and research experience of the physiologist for the sake of perspective and a basis for comparison of the academic and research backgrounds of the two men.

James Macleod was born in Cluny, near Dunkeld in Scotland on September 6, 1876. An excellent student, Macleod attended Aberdeen University where the records show that he won first prize in all his first year subjects and graduated with "Honourable Distinction" and M.B.Ch.B. in 1898. The following year he was awarded a travelling fellowship and studied in the historic Physiologic Institute in Leipzig which counts amongst its illustrious alumni the distinguished philosopher Goethe, musicians Robert Schumann and Richard Wagner as well as the German Chancellor Angela Merkel.

The following year 1899, Macleod returned to England to continue studies in physiology at the London Hospital. Within three years he was promoted to Lecturer in Biochemistry. He was there till 1903 when he was appointed Professor of Physiology at Western Reserve University in Cleveland, Ohio. He was 27 years old.

As far back as 1905 Macleod had been interested not only in carbohydrate metabolism but in diabetes.

His early interest in carbohydrate metabolism had resulted in a book, *Diabetes: Its Pathological Physiology* by John J. R. Macleod, M. B., Ch. B., D. P. H. Professor of Physiology Western Reserve University, Cleveland, Ohio, USA. Late Demonstrator of Physiology, London Hospital.

The book had been published in London and also in New York where the prestigious firm of Longmans, Green & Co had released it in 1913. Macleod had also published over 40 papers on carbohydrate metabolism and experimental diabetes.

He was familiar with von Mering's and Minkowski's work published in 1889. In 1908 he had also conducted an experiment to investigate the possibility of the brain causing the blood glucose levels to rise, a cardinal feature of diabetes. However, like many workers in the field, although Macleod believed the pancreas was the organ involved – the "seat" of diabetes – he, like other workers in the field, had not been able to demonstrate the exact role of the pancreas in diabetes.

Macleod was aware of the suggestion by Laguesse in 1893 that the islets of Langerhans possibly produced an internal secretion. He also knew that Sharpey-Schaeffer in 1916 had named the secretion "insuline". It must be emphasised that at the time "insuline" was still a hypothetical substance.

In 1918 he was elected Professor Physiology at University of Toronto, Canada. He was at the same time appointed the Director of Physiological Laboratory and Dean of the Faculty of Medicine at the University of Toronto

At the time of his first meeting with Frederick Banting in November 1920, Macleod was 42 years old. He was a physiologist with an established international reputation with nearly 2 decades of research experience and was a recognised authority on carbohydrate metabolism. He had published extensively on various aspects of carbohydrate metabolism. He had also written a book,

Physiology and Biochemistry in Modern Medicine, which at that time was in its third edition.

In short, Macleod's faultless academic record, post graduate studies and experience in physiology, were in a different sphere from the 30-year-old journeyman surgeon who had been a co-author of a lone journal article and had never achieved or been awarded a single academic honour. Yet here he was sitting opposite Macleod in his office on that fateful morning of November 8, 1920.

Obviously Macleod had little in common with the stranger facing him in his office on that wintry November morning.

Given the gap in the knowledge of physiology in general and the subject of insulin in particular, the aligning of the stars with the accomplished physiologist and the army surgeon was decidedly a meeting of opposites from the start to, unfortunately, the end of the association. At the conclusion of Banting's appeal to Macleod, the latter gave qualified approval for the project to be carried out in his department.

None of the three, Macleod, Banting and Best had little in common other than an academic association.

Neither would any of them have had any inkling that this casual and unplanned assignment would link forever their destinies in medical folklore.

JAMES BERTRAM COLLIP (1892–1965)

The fourth member who joined the team towards the end of 1921 was by far the most intellectually gifted. Born in Belleville Ontario in 1892 Collip had humble beginnings. His parents, James Dennis Collip and Mahala Frances Vance Collip ran a florist shop. His early education was in the one–room school house in Belleville before going to Belleville High School until 1908 when at the age of 15 he gained admission to Trinity College in Toronto where he met his future wife Ray Vivian Ralph. At age 15 he was considered too young to enter medical school. Collip enrolled in a biochemistry course and in 1916 gained a PhD. He was 24 years old. Even before he had completed his doctorate, he was offered the position of Lecturer in Biochemistry at the University of Alberta in Edmonton in 1915. Collip was to remain in Alberta for 13 years.

A prodigious worker, Collip spent his summer months conducting research in various fields of biochemistry. This took him not only to other research centres in Canada but also to research laboratories in the United States. He had spent time at the University of Chicago and then in Great Britain in Sheffield.

In April, 1921 a Rockefeller Travelling Fellowship brought Collip back to the University of Toronto to conduct research in the Department of Physiological Chemistry. The head of the department was James Macleod. This was the beginning of Collip's role in the insulin story.

Thus in terms of experience in research as well as qualifications it is clear that Collip was in a different class from the two fellow-researchers namely Banting and Best.

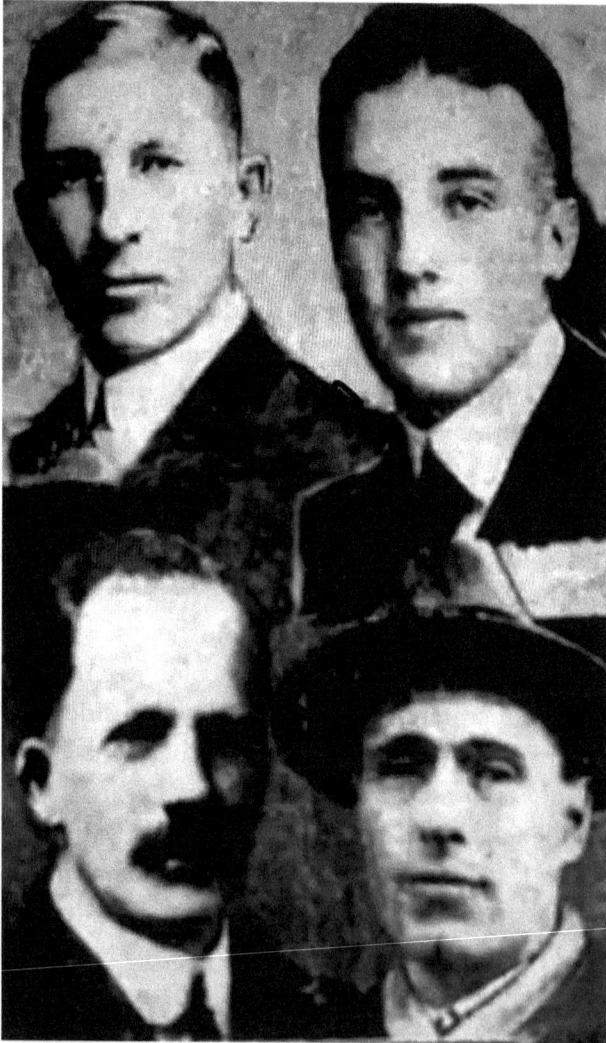

Insulin team. (clockwise from top left) Banting, Best, Collip, Macleod.

The Spark Which Ignited the Flame

As part of his teaching duties at Western University, Banting had to give lectures to medical students. Indeed it was his first task every week which began with a lecture to the students on Monday morning. As it turned out, it was a Monday morning assignment which led to the most important event in the young Torontonian's life.

The last weekend of October 1920 had been emotional, even traumatic for Banting. Just before reporting for military duties on 19 March 1917, he had become engaged to Edith Roach. On his return however, he discovered that her feelings for him had changed. She was decidedly cooler, not the ardent sweetheart she had been at their parting. Possibly she was having second thoughts after seeing the changes in him: a tendency to swear, heavy drinking and his new habit of chain – smoking.

According to papers held in the Banting House NHSC archives, a letter from Banting's sister Essie expressed her reservations about Edith's suitability as "to really be a partner..... So perhaps fate is just intervening before it is too late and showing you both that a mistake has been made."

So Banting would hardly have been in a stable frame of mind when preparing the lecture to be delivered on the following morning, Monday, to his students.

On the last Sunday in October 1920 Banting prepared a lecture on carbohydrate metabolism to be given to the students on the following morning. He did not have any particular interest in carbohydrate metabolism in general or diabetes in particular. It was simply a subject in the syllabus he was teaching the students. It is doubtful if he had had any experience in diabetes. In later years he commented that one of his classmates, Joe Gilchrist had suffered from diabetes. Banting had never treated anyone with the condition.

Having completed his preparation for the lecture, the unhappy rejected suitor retired to bed with a copy of his recently delivered November issue of the journal "*Surgery, Gynaecology and Obstetrics.*"

Fred Banting would hardly have been in a stable frame of mind when preparing the lecture to be delivered on the following morning to his students.

An article with the title "The Relation of the Islets of Langerhans to Diabetes with Special Reference to Cases of Pancreatic Lithiasis," by Moses Barron attracted Banting's attention since he was going to be talking about carbohydrate metabolism the next day.

Many years later Banting recounted the story in his memoir, *The Story of Insulin* published in 1940:

"I was disturbed and could not sleep. I thought about the lecture and about the article and I thought about my miseries and how I would like to get out of debt and away from worry.

Finally about two in the morning, after the lecture and the article had been chasing each other through my mind for some time, the idea occurred to me that by experimental ligation of the duct and subsequent degradation of a portion of the pancreas, one might obtain the internal secretion free from the external secretion. I got up and wrote down the idea and spent most of the night thinking about it."

Bliss, with access to Banting's notebook housed in the Academy of Medicine in Toronto reproduced the notes in his book *The Discovery of Insulin.*

"Diabetus" (*sic*).

"Ligate pancreatic duct of dog. Keep dogs alive till acini degenerate leaving islets.

Try to isolate the internal secretion of these to relieve glycosuria."

The role of the islets of Langerhans as a cause of diabetes was at this stage just a hypothesis and Moses Barron, the writer of the article, did not in anyway emphasise the findings, merely presenting them as one more piece of evidence worthy of consideration in the search for the cause of diabetes.

Banting's reaction to the article, however, was entirely different from Barron's. This is confirmed in a personal letter Barron wrote to Banting in February, 1923. Parts of Barron's letter are reproduced below.*

However the credit is divided, and it seems to be apportioned differently by just about everyone with an opinion on the subject, it is difficult to escape the fact that Banting, in spite of all his shortcomings, was the first investigator to pursue the isolation of the elusive secretion believing that this could settle the question of the cause of diabetes.

There had been limited discussion on this subject following the dramatic demonstration of the pancreas as the "seat" of diabetes by none other than Oskar Minkowski. Often regarded as the most brilliant medical scholar of his generation, Minkowski did not regard the shrivelled remnant of the pancreas which was left after the organ had been destroyed by blocking the pancreatic duct as having any bearing on diabetes.

Barron says,

"I assure you that I feel I am flattered by that reference and it was very kind of you indeed to make mention of that article in your address. Although I was quite interested in the study of the pancreas at the time when I published that article, *I did not have the faintest idea or hope that it would be at any time or in any way be sufficiently suggestive to start such an epoch-making investigation as you have undertaken......*

......I feel it an honour to be in anyway mentioned in connection with this work of yours, and I wish that I had actually had some real part in the investigation. I wish you and your co-workers great success in furthering the refinement of the insulin and of bringing it's manufacture to a stage where it will be within reach of the million or more of suffering humanity in America alone who are crying for a relief....."

---

* The manually typed letter signed by Moses Barron dated February 14, 1923 is quoted here in part. (I have typed the relevant part in italics).

Barron, born in Russia had come to the United States with his parents when he was five years old. He had studied medicine at the University of Minnesota and after the First World War was working as a pathologist when he wrote the article.

While doing an autopsy, Barron was intrigued to find a single stone completely blocking the pancreatic duct. When he examined the pancreas under the microscope (as Paul Langerhans had done many years earlier), he found that the cells producing the digestive enzyme had been destroyed but the cells of the islets had not been affected. Barron was intrigued when on inspecting the specimen from his own case to discover that the changes at autopsy were the same as had been reported by researchers who had blocked the (pancreatic) duct by tying it off.

He saw his work as another piece in the mosaic of findings, hypotheses, suggestions and speculations on the underlying cause of diabetes. He said as much in a personal letter to Banting after the latter's success in isolating the secretion of the islet cells.

Banting's Dilemma

Given Banting's background of medical education – medical school followed by hospital training shortened by war service (even though he had studied and succeeded in the examinations to gain Membership to the English College of Surgeons) his experience in treating patients had mostly been during the war and had mostly consisted of attending to war injuries. This was hardly a qualification for an academic career or medical research.

At a loss for which direction to take, he did what many medical graduates do. He went to Western's library. Needless to say he came away empty-handed. One can only speculate on what information he would have sought on how to proceed and where he would have looked.

His next port of call was the Head of the department, Professor F.O. Miller who, as already mentioned, was Professor of Physiology at Western. Miller was familiar with the research facilities in different universities in Canada having himself been engaged in medical research over many years. Unfortunately he was a neurophysiologist and rightly admitted to having virtually no knowledge of carbohydrate metabolism.

Still Banting would not give up. He asked Miller if there was an institution nearby which would consider a new project to explore his idea. Again he failed. Miller explained to the aspiring researcher that for his project he would need to find a research laboratory which had facilities for housing large animals like dogs. Dogs were being used in the kind of experiment Banting was contemplating. Western just did not have such facilities.

Miller's long experience as a teacher and researcher had repeatedly shown him how easily aspiring young researchers were discouraged. He hastened to tell Banting that his idea was promising but felt compelled to warn the young man of failure and also of the likelihood of the project having been tried before by someone else.

However Miller had underestimated Banting's dogged determination. To the returned soldier and winner of the. Military Cross, these rejections paled in comparison with the rejection by Edith only a day or so earlier.

If anything, Miller's reservations increased Banting's resolve.

Then Miller made one more suggestion. He had heard of a professor of physiology who had previously been in the United States and was now in Toronto. Miller recalled this professor's interest in carbohydrate research and advised Banting to talk to him.

Frederick Banting meets Professor James Macleod May 15, 1921

If Miller's caution had caused Banting to hesitate, the hesitation didn't last long. Within 24 hours of hearing about the professor Banting had telephoned Macleod.

A letter dated March 11, 1921 from Macleod to Banting to confirm the appointment is important because it records details of the arrangement, particularly the limitations such as in the number of staff available to help in the care of the experimental animals (dogs). The letter said,

"Dear Dr. Banting,

I will be glad to have you come up here on May 15th as you suggest, and see what you can do with the problem of Pancreatic Diabetes, which we spoke about. I doubt, however, whether it would be advisable to attempt any preliminary operations during the Easter holidays, since between that time and May 18th there will be no one here personally interested in the supervision of the animals, and this supervision, as you know is of extreme importance in all researches of this character. Between these dates, everyone and the staff in the laboratory, will be under the unfortunate necessity of devoting a great part of his time to examinations, detail and to other things pertaining to the winding up of the session. I think that after May 15th. when you could get close personal attention to the work, it could proceed satisfactorily within the time you suggest you could give to it.

With regards,
I am
Sincerely yours
J.J.R. Macleod (Signed by hand).

Thus, within a week of hearing about the physiologist, the aspiring researcher had secured an appointment with the Toronto professor and on the appointed day was sitting opposite Professor John James Rickard Macleod in the professor's office in the Department of Physiology at the University of Toronto.

It was also only weeks since his heartbreaking rejection by Edith Roach but the decorated First World War veteran had scant regard for omens.

The sequence of events described above also reveals one of the character traits in Banting which I noticed from the time I started my preparation for this project. His capacity for acting on an idea with a minimum of fuss or vacillation will be seen again and again. To his supporters this was considered an indication of his dedication and drive. To his critics however his tendency to charge ahead regardless of the consequences represented a disregard verging on disrespect towards any who opposed his views. At this time the figure of authority first and foremost was James Macleod the professor of the department and head of the laboratory where Banting was working. Unfortunately Banting's habit of upsetting those in authority increased during the months of summer in 1921 when he was carrying out the experiments in his pursuit of the elusive secretion.

It is important to appreciate that in addition to the position of Head of the Department of Physiology, Macleod was also the Dean of the Faculty of Medicine at Toronto University. The role of the Dean in the university is an important and prestigious position given to a member on the staff who is recognised for his qualities of leadership and competence. The Dean is responsible not only for academic progress but also general administration including fiscal matters. Therefore if Macleod reminded Banting of the authority he had not only in the matter concerning Banting but in all such endeavours within that institution, he was merely stating a fact which he was certain was not known to the aspiring and enthusiastic researcher sitting opposite.

Macleod's agreement was qualified and the possibility of failure had been couched in the phrase "It was worth trying" and "negative results would be of great physiological value." The message was not lost on Banting.

Discouraged, he sought the advice of his former supervisor Clarence L. Starr, the highly respected chief surgeon of the Hospital for Sick Children in Toronto. Starr had become a "medical father-figure" to Banting.

Starr rang Macleod who expressed reservations pointing out to the senior surgeon Banting's limited experience and qualifications. He may have been comparing Banting's postgraduate career with his own. Starr passed this on to Banting and advised that it would be wise for him not to give up his current paying position. He also mentioned Macleod's suggestion that Banting "might possibly come in the summer and put in a month or two then."

Heeding Starr's advice Banting returned to his London Ontario lodgings to spend the rest of winter there. However try as he might the thought of pursuing the isolation of the pancreatic extract would not go away.

According to Bliss, Banting "read widely on the subject of carbohydrate metabolism and even read a little about diabetes."

It is clear that Macleod could see possible value in Banting's proposition which if successful, would isolate the product of the islets by ligating the pancreatic duct. This had not been done successfully previously. Therefore Macleod considered the project to be worthy of a trial.

Lastly, as will be described later, Macleod provided practical assistance without which Banting, who had no background or experience in research, would not have been able to accomplish this goal.

In short, it could be argued that without Macleod's guidance and at times participation, the insulin project in Toronto, if left entirely in Banting's hands, may well have floundered.

Although Banting was a surgeon it must be remembered that removal of the entire pancreas was still a hazardous operation. The organ has a rich blood supply and unless each artery is tied off, catastrophic haemorrhaging floods the abdomen and the patient dies. Years earlier Claude Bernard had stated that this operation was not possible without causing death of the patient. Much of Banting's surgical experience was obtained during the war when the majority of surgical procedures consisted of repairing shrapnel wounds. Little wonder that Macleod, clearly apprehensive about Banting undertaking this operation chose to assist him when the first animal was operated on. Minkowski's successful removal of the pancreas over 30 years before Banting is another reminder of the extraordinary capability and dexterity of the European master. Dramatic and remarkable as the success of that operation clearly was, it could be argued that Minkowski's presence of mind in correlating the frequent passage of urine with the possibility of diabetes which led him to test the urine for glucose was the critical step which led subsequent investigators in the right direction in their search for insulin.

Minkowski had narrowed the field to where the elusive substance central to the cause of diabetes was located.

It was the pancreas.

That this was the beginning of the journey undertaken in a country far removed from the well-known cradles of medical knowledge and research and which culminated in the isolation of insulin is now part of the history of medicine. It also has pride of place in the treatment of diabetes.

Finally, it must not be forgotten that the name of Toronto, the city where the experiments took place has also etched its name in the annals of the history of medical experimentation and life-saving and life-changing discoveries.

In attributing credit to Banting it is important to note that he had firstly, recognised the possibility of the internal secretion being within the pancreas and, after tying off the duct, had succeeded in overcoming the difficulty all previous workers had encountered in separating the extract of the islets of Langerhans. He was then able to demonstrate that this extract lowered the level of glucose (sugar) in the experimental diabetes he had produced in dogs. This was the critical difference between earlier attempts and the Torontonian's successful experiments.

It must be acknowledged that the essence of Banting's contribution to the discovery of insulin lay in his proven capacity to see or at least sense, then doggedly pursue, the essential steps missed by others. Where the earlier workers had stopped when the pancreas was discovered to be the seat of diabetes by von Mering and Minkowski, Banting, after reading the Barron article, assiduously pursued the pancreatic remnant which was left after the destruction of the digestive body of the gland.

Nor did his early failures deter him.

The First Idea

This is best described in the words of Banting and Best and is taken from their paper which was published in the Journal of Laboratory and Clinical Medicine in February 1922. It also includes information which flies in the face of popular misconceptions held in some quarters relating to the relative contributions of different members of the wider team engaged in finding insulin.

"The hypothesis underlying this series of experiments was first formulated by one of us in November, 1920, while reading an article* dealing with the relation of the isles (sic) of Langerhans to diabetes. From the passage in the article, which gives a resume of degenerative changes in the acini of the pancreas, following ligation of the duct, the idea presented itself that since the acinous, but not the islet tissue, degenerates after this operation, advantage might be taken of this fact to prepare an active extract of islet tissue. The subsidiary hypothesis was the trypsinogen or its derivatives were antagonistic to the internal secretion of the gland. The failures of other investigators in this much–worked field were thus accounted for.

The feasibility of the hypothesis having been recognised by Professor G.J.R. Macleod, work was begun under his direction in February 1921, in the physiological laboratory of the University of Toronto. Help was also generously rendered by Professors Henderson, Fitzgerald, Graham, and Defries."

Early Challenges for Banting and Best

The essential steps in the story of insulin were firstly its discovery followed by the refinements which were needed to make it suitable for use in the treatment of diabetes, and finally, it's manufacture to make it available to the suffering and their carers. This train of events can be thought of as the three Ds of the insulin story namely: discovery, development and delivery.

---

* The article referred to was in the November issue of the journal *"Surgery Gynaecology and Obstetrics."*

It must be remembered that the role of the Islets of Langerhans as a cause of diabetes at this time was just a hypothesis and Banting did not emphasise the fact but merely presented it as one more piece of evidence to be considered in the search for the cause of diabetes.

Progress was slow in the early weeks for several reasons. To start with, neither Banting nor Best had any practical experience in producing diabetes in an experimental animal. So the first exercise was to search the literature for a method for turning normal dogs into diabetic animals. This initiative proved challenging because much of the research work on diabetes had been carried out in Germany and France and the pertinent information was to be found only in German and French scientific journals and publications. Neither of the aspiring researchers knew German. As for the knowledge of French, in spite of the French presence in Canada since the early days of European immigration into the country, neither of the Torontonians, each of whom was a descendent of English immigrants, possessed even a working knowledge of French let alone the technical/scientific terminology employed in French medical journals. These deficiencies were to have some unfortunate consequences for both of them at a later time on their scientific journey.

Curiously, there is no record of either of the Torontonians looking for information closer to home. In early 1913 Frederick M. Allen had published "Glycosuria and Diabetes" which had been released for sale by Harvard University Press of Cambridge Massachusetts. Two pieces of information in this tome which would have been of assistance to the fledgeling researchers were firstly, exhaustive review of the literature – the volume of 1179 pages contained more than 1200 references – as well as details of Allen's own experiments. Between 1909 and 1912 he had operated on hundreds of animals in his laboratory to remove the pancreas which made the animals diabetic. He had operated on 200 dogs, 200 cats and a smaller number of rabbits, guinea pigs and rats.

Allen had recorded and catalogued his methodology in meticulous detail.

The fact that neither Banting nor Best was aware of this publication is curious to say the least. Equally surprising is that Macleod with his background of knowledge and record of publications including a book on diabetes mentioned above, did not offer the obvious suggestion in this regard. Later, after several months of experimentation including the surgical removal of the pancreas from dogs, Banting discovered Allen's method and wrote in one of his notebooks that he had used the method described by the American diabetes specialist.

This is not the only instance where the absence of much needed advice and assistance from the head of the department in which the experiments were carried out by the two researchers on insulin raises obvious questions on just how involved James Macleod was in the search for insulin.

Compounding the difficulties for Banting was a lack of funds. As far as Best was concerned, Macleod had told him at the outset that he could work with Banting in the department during his summer holidays but there was "no stipend."

Banting loaned Best money to cover living expenses. Clearly the puritan ethics of thrift and hard work applied as much to Best even though he came from the well-to-do family of a highly respected general practitioner, Dr Herbert Best.

Little in the way of experiments was done in the first few weeks of June which was particularly frustrating for Banting. He made little headway. As was typical, he became angry and impatient. He blamed Best for his own failure to get results and, like the proverbial bad workman, blamed the lack of scientific equipment. He also said the equipment had not been cleaned properly, a lapse for which Banting blamed Best. Best had been away in militia camp for 10 days at the end of June.

An amusing detail contained in the Best family papers speaks of the young man spending most of his time at the militia camp riding horses which were difficult to ride for the others in the camp. Best was known for his proficiency in horsemanship.

To his credit, Best on his return to the laboratory, took the senior man's "severe talking to" in good grace and immediately proceeded to remedy all the ills which had led to Banting's rants. He spent the rest of the day, then continued through the whole night scrubbing the laboratory bench and cleaning the glassware.

Little is written about this but clearly Banting was taken by the young man's many qualities especially his humility and capacity for hard work, to say nothing of his academic prowess. Best had joined Banting immediately after completing his university course from which he had graduated with honours and had come second in his class.

The animals chosen for the experiments were dogs which had been the choice from the beginning of the pursuit for the cause of diabetes. Minkowski had carried out his experiments on dogs. Later, experiments on the well-publicised – and photographed – dogs were used by the French physiologist Eduard Hedon. Macleod had provided a few dogs for the initial part of the experiments but later when they had run out of the initial pack of the animals assigned by Macleod, there were unconfirmed reports of the two researchers buying strays or abandoned dogs from the neighbourhood.

The Brown Dog Affair

Medical research using animals, especially larger animals like dogs, remains controversial to this day. The work by Hedon which involved removing the pancreas from dogs was done after the "brown dog affair." The name arose after a statue had been commissioned in memory of a brown dog which had died after medical experimentation. Antivivisectionists had erected the statue in London's Battersea Park. News of the dog's death resulted in riots and a group of medical students tore down the statue and threw it in the river Thames.

The "laboratory" assigned to Banting by Macleod was a small, poorly ventilated room situated right next to the smelly dog kennels. In spite of the poor conditions in the medical building where they worked, the two frequently spent the whole day and night in the oppressive heat and humidity typical of summers in Toronto.

The first part of the exercise consisted of essentially two steps. Firstly one dog was subjected to removal of the pancreas. This produced diabetes in the animal.

Next, four or five dogs would undergo operations to have the pancreatic duct tied off. Their wounds would be sutured and dressed and the animals would be returned to the kennels. In these the pancreas would be destroyed as a result of the pancreatic duct being tied off. It had been shown by Barron that not all the material of the pancreas was destroyed. That which remained contained the small nests of cells described by the German medical student Paul Langerhans in 1869. This was the material which remained within the shrivelled pancreas after most of the gland had been destroyed because of the strongly acidic digestive juices which had been stopped from escaping the gland after the duct had been tied off. It usually took 4 to 6 weeks for this to happen.

At that time the dogs were operated on once again and the shrivelled pancreas was removed. The pancreatic remnants were then crushed and mixed with various liquids to make an extract. The extract was then injected into the diabetic dog to see if it caused it's blood sugar to fall. High blood sugar levels are the critical abnormality in diabetes not only in laboratory animals but in the men, women and children afflicted by this condition.

With hindsight, it is a wonder that this simple reasoning used by Banting had escaped previous workers including many highly respected physicians and scientists like Naunyn in Germany and Bouchardat in France who had spent many years of their working lives treating patients with diabetes and studying the condition. Both had written books on the subject.

The renowned physiologist Oskar Minkowski had tried to produce an extract from the pancreas to reduce urinary sugar but had not succeeded in doing so.

July remained oppressive but Banting was uncompromising in his pursuit and proceeded along the lines outlined above. He removed the pancreas of 4 or five dogs to make them diabetic. The exact number is unclear as he was not overly concerned with note-taking, a habit which was going to have unfortunate consequences. The second part of the experiment was to operate on a single dog by tying off it's pancreatic duct. After 4 to 6 weeks the bulk of the pancreas was destroyed leaving the remains which, after reading Barron's article, Banting left intact the nest of cells namely the islets suspected of being the reason for the animal not becoming diabetic. Therefore the next step was to make an extract from the shrivelled pancreatic remnants containing the islets.

Then if, as Banting believed or hoped, the hypothesis was correct, injecting the extract into a diabetic dog would reduce the level of blood sugar.

On July 30, 1921 the extract from a diabetic dog number 410 was, for the first time, shown to have this effect.

For Banting and Best this was success and a reason for unbridled joy and excitement. However they realised that the strict rules of scientific experimentation would pay little attention to a single result which is often dismissed as "an isolated finding."

More than one dog would need to be benefited in this way before any claims could be made. Banting realised that a bigger test was to convince the head of the department, Professor James Macleod.

On August 3, 2021 dog number 408 was made diabetic by a different technique. The previous dog, on the advice of Professor Macleod had the pancreas removed according to the two-stage operation used by the French physiologist mentioned above, Eduard Hedon. At Best's suggestion Banting attempted the removal of dog 408's pancreas in a single operation. He found this to be a much easier method and more importantly, the dog survived the procedure.

Injection with the extract in this dog once again lowered the blood sugar, this time not for one day but for four days.

Unfortunately the researchers' joy was short-lived. Three days after the operation, on August 7, the dog died.

However the fact that the extract had kept the blood sugar down for four days convinced the researchers that they were on the right track. They reflected on the many dogs they had lost prior to getting the results they wanted in these two animals.

As a gift to mark the end of my Fellowship in 1970, Leo Krall gave me a highly valued photograph. It was the page from the notebook of Banting and Best which recorded the dramatic results of the experiment on 7 August 1921. It detailed for the first time the falling levels of blood sugar in the experimental animal, a dog, which had developed diabetes after removal of its pancreas by the surgeon, Frederick Banting, assisted by his student helper, Charles Best. The experiment had proceeded throughout the night, and the blood sugar recordings were made at 1 am, 2 am, 3 am and 4 am following injections of the extract. With each injection the blood sugar value had fallen. This was the critical experiment which showed that the extract made from the insulin-producing cells in the pancreas could control blood sugar in a diabetic animal.

The death of dog 408 distressed Banting even more than the many dogs he had lost earlier in whom the extract had not been effective. With his surgical background Banting was convinced that the main reason for the infection lay in the poor operating conditions. His work on human patients as a young surgeon including his time in the army where much of the surgery consisted of cleaning up and suturing wounds was always done in conditions of – in medical jargon –"strict asepsis." Operating on animals required the same degree of cleanliness or "sterility."

He remembered the often-quoted Latin aphorism "Mortui vivos docent" (the dead teach the living), and the emphasis in his surgery tutorials on post-mortem examination of patients when the cause of death was unclear.

At autopsy on dog 408 Banting was dismayed to find widespread infection in the animal. He had suspected this, given the poor operating conditions in the facilities provided by the department.

Banting appealed to his mentor Dr. Starr, the Chief Surgeon at Toronto General Hospital. Starr was appalled. Immediate arrangements were made for the dogs to be operated on in a proper surgical facility within the hospital.

The second matter which concerned him was the process/s involved in the preparation of the extract. The variable effects on the blood glucose of the experimental animals made him wonder whether the extracts were of uniform quality. Early in the course of his discussions with Macleod Banting had met a biochemist by the name of J.B. Collip who was visiting Toronto on a travelling fellowship and had expressed an interest in joining him. Macleod had discouraged this but Banting decided that he would raise the subject again. He had remembered that Collip had a reputation for an expertise in preparing extracts.

Returning to the story of dog 408, both Banting and Best wrote to Macleod, who had gone on holidays, telling him of their success as well as their concerns over the infections and the need for improved facilities. In the same letter Banting emphasised the qualities of his younger associate and according to the Best family records said, "Best has taught me the chemistry so that we work together all the time and check up on each other's readings". He also told Macleod that Best wanted to continue to work with him.

Macleod in his reply dated August 23, 1921 had been positive and encouraging but, as is common in an experienced researcher, also cautious.

He said "....your results are definitely positive, but it is not absolutely certain.....

You know that if you can prove *to the satisfaction of everyone* that such extracts really have the power to reduce blood sugar in pancreatic diabetes, you would have achieved a very great deal. Kleiner and others who have published somewhat similar results have not convinced others because their proofs were not adequate. It's very easy often in science to satisfy ones own self about some point but it's very hard to build up the stronghold of proof which others cannot pull down. Now, for example, supposing I wanted to be one of those critics I would say that your results on dog 408 were not absolutely convincing..."

Here Macleod was referring to the death of dog 408. A macabre comment often heard in scientific discourse is, "the experiment was a success but the patient died."

Regardless of the effect of the extract on the dog, its death overshadowed all other aspects of the experiment. This left just one experimental animal in which the extract had lowered the blood glucose level.

One of Macleod's favourite expressions when discussing results of scientific exercises was "One result is no result."

Best in his letter had mentioned the use of "two depancreatised dogs side by side, only one receiving injections of extract".

Including two dogs in their research is a crucial requirement in such experiments. The use of a "control" subject paired with a "test" subject described in a letter by Best to his fiancé Margaret Mahon is important because it shows that the experiments were carried out according to the design of the two investigators and not at the suggestion or recommendations of Macleod because at the time of these experiments the professor was still on his summer holidays in Scotland.

Best had written "we are doing identical operations on dogs. We are going to give one the extract and the other none and study the condition of each. It will be quite a crucial* test for "Isletin." In scientific parlance the dog getting the extract is the "test" subject while the one getting no extract is the "control".

(Isletin was the term used by Banting and Best for the extract).

---

* Crucial indeed, because without a control such an experiment would not get past first base in any scientific establishment let alone where, it was hoped, that the project if successful would eventually be tried on diabetics.

Given the rapidity of the sequence of events starting with Banting's idea and it's progression to the first promising results from experimentation, a time-line of the salient events is helpful in keeping track of the insulin story as it unfolds.

TIMELINE OF BANTING'S EXPERIMENTS IN THE DISCOVERY OF INSULIN

October 31, 1920: Banting's bedtime reading provides idea.

November 1, 1920: Banting approaches Professor Miller.

November 7, 1920: Banting meets Professor Macleod.

April 1921: Macleod assigns Charles Best to assist Banting.

May 16, 1921: Start of project.

May17,1921: Macleod joins Banting and Best-first experiment.

Mid June 1921: Macleod leaves for summer holidays in Scotland.

July 30, 1921: dog 410, the first successful injection.

August 3, 1921: Banting changes his surgical technique of the two – stage operation to remove the pancreas as pioneered by Eduard Hedon and, removes the whole pancreas in one operation.

Dog 408 : extract lowers dog's blood glucose for four days but dog dies.

August 9, 1921: researchers report their success to Macleod.

August 11, 1921:"Five operations in one day to treat more than one dog."

August 15, 1921: The control experiment. Dog 92 given extract at midnight. Dog 409 not treated ("control"). Dog 92 thrives, dog 409 dies.

November 14, 1921: results discussed at physiology journal club. Professor Taylor suggests a "longevity experiment."

November 18, 1921: longevity experiment started on dog 33, Marjorie.

December 6, 1921 Marjorie treated with extract and blood sugar remains well controlled for 70 days.

December 12, 1921: Banting and Best experiment successfully on dog 35 with extract from bovine pancreas.

Mid-December 1921: J. B. Collip joins researchers to start next (development) phase.

An interesting part of this story is the role of Macleod. Opinions regarding his contributions vary. It is clear that there was an element of dissatisfaction, even hostility, on the part of Banting towards the physiologist but in fairness it should be observed that were it not for Macleod's assistance it is doubtful if Banting would have achieved what he did – at least not in Toronto.

Regardless of the adequacy of, or the willingness or otherwise with which they were given the various contributions of Macleod must not be forgotten. He did provide Banting with the facilities for the work to be carried out and assigned one of his students, Charles Best as assistant. Assigning a student to help with various tasks such as giving tutorials to students in the lower years of the course or helping with a project being conducted in the laboratory by a senior researcher was common practice. It allowed students in the medical, physiology or science faculties to gain an insight into some of the practical aspects of research. It was also a way of them earning pocket money as many of them were forever short of cash. Having someone on hand to attend to chores like cleaning the equipment and the bench, running errands and attending to animals freed the researchers to concentrate on the essentials of the project. Usually additional help was given when animals were being used. For Banting's work Macleod allowed only one helper, Best.

A timeline of Macleod's movements during the critical period when the work which culminated in the discovery of insulin was done helps to provide a perspective on some of the controversies involving him.

Timeline of Macleod's Summer Holidays in 1921

May 17, 1921: Macleod assigns Best to assist Banting.
Mid June, 1921: leaves for annual holidays in Scotland.
August 9, 1921: letters from Banting and Best to Macleod.
August 23, 1921: Macleod replies to the letters.
September 21, 1921: Macleod returns to work.

Banting and Best continued their work after hearing from Macleod and proceeded to carry out the "control" experiment mentioned above.

On August 11, 1921 they removed the pancreas from two dogs, number 92 and 409.

Dog 92, a yellow collie was treated with the extract. Dog 409, the control, was not treated.

Within 48 hours the yellow collie was active and "in fine spirits."The control dog 409 was barely able to walk.

On August 15, the control dog died. Dog 92, the yellow collie was thriving and had become the laboratory's pet.

A week later when Banting used, as a trial, an extract made from the pancreas of a cat on dog 92, the favourite collie went into profound shock and after lingering for nine days, died on August 31. Banting wept.

This was essentially the end of their first series of experiments. Although a few experiments were done during the latter part of August and in September, Banting and Best felt that their summer's work was essentially over. They made no plans for any further experiments before Professor Macleod arrived back in Toronto on September 21, 1921 at the end of his summer holidays.

Banting's relationship with Macleod

Much has been made of clashes between Banting and Macleod. Their disagreements have been attributed to the personalities of the two men. However, factual accounts of the discovery of insulin include several examples of lack of guidance or supervision by the head of the department which claimed credit for discovering insulin on the basis of the work having been done in that institution. The actual studies and experiments were carried out by Banting with Best's assistance. In fact the bulk of the investigative work which culminated in the isolation of an effective albeit imperfect insulin extract was completed in Macleod's absence. Such omissions are perhaps of greater importance in assigning credit for the work on insulin rather than the clash of different personalities in the group. Interpersonal difficulties are encountered in many fields of studies and experiments.

The euphoria of their initial success prior to Macleod's return from his summer holidays was, in Banting's case, tempered by his own precarious financial position. In August, 1921 in conversation with Velyien Henderson, the professor of pharmacology, Banting had told him of his lack of funds. As was Banting's habit, he often used his charm on the secretaries of professors to get an appointment. In this case it was a woman called Jean Orr. She recalled a conversation with Banting some 60 years later saying that he had emptied his pocket of coins which added up to 7 cents and had declared to the embarrassed young woman that the sum was all the money had to live on "If I don't get a job."

Henderson who had developed a liking for Banting had hinted that he might be able to help and had written to the president of the university about the young man's difficulties.

Banting and Best met with Macleod on his return in late September. Banting asked for an improvement in their working conditions which had made the summer of '21 such a trial. He requested repairs to the floor of the operating room, a boy to look after the dogs, better working space − a new room if possible, and a salary.

Although Macleod had promised assistance in the letter he had written to Banting and Best during his holidays he seemed reluctant to honour the undertakings he had given. There were several reasons for his change of heart. A new building was already in advanced planning stages, the researchers had gone through more dogs than planned, and Macleod was concerned that further expenditure on the insulin project would compromise the department's capacity for financing other work. Macleod had not disclosed to Banting and Best that even before allocating the few dogs for their project the department had already used more than 380 dogs on various experiments.

As Dean of the Faculty he was also concerned about the arrangement, made in his absence and without consultation, for operations on animals from the university's laboratories to be carried out in the hospital facilities normally reserved for treating human subjects. One reason for this was that the location of the physiology department was across the road from the hospital which meant that the animals were being carried in full view of the public thus raising the possibility of being reported to and antagonising, the powerful antivivisectionist lobby in Toronto. In a tactical manoeuvre Macleod, shortly after hearing of this arrangement, set up the Surgical Research Committee which was to make the final decision on whether to permit or disallow a proposed animal experiment to be carried out at the University. Banting had secured the approval of the committee to continue his animal experiments.

As far as Banting was concerned this change of mind by Macleod was breaking a promise. Given his volatile temper the resulting confrontation with Macleod was inevitable.

A dramatic version of this confrontation is contained in the book by Michael Bliss. The details have been derived mainly from information contained in the Best family archives. There is considerable variation in the account as recounted by Charles Best depending on his audience. For example the account given to Henry Dale by Best is far less colourful than the one contained in Michael Bliss's book. According to Henry Best, Bliss had visited Charles Best's widow on at least three occasions. The details add little to the well known difficulties which existed between Banting and Macleod.

As far as the story of the discovery of insulin is concerned, suffice it to say that after this the already frosty relations between Macleod and Banting remained at best cool and at worst hostile for the rest of their association and only ended in1928 when Macleod returned to Aberdeen at the end of his tenure in Toronto.

Macleod Takes Charge

Regardless of the reservations, even criticism which may be levelled at Banting and Best for jumping to premature conclusions as far as the discovery of insulin was concerned the fact remains that the two researchers had seen, recognised and documented the fall in the blood glucose levels of two dogs when they had injected the animals with the extract prepared from the pancreatic remnants. No one could, or for that matter did, dispute this fact. Banting and Best were convinced that they had discovered insulin through the experiments conducted that summer. As noted previously, the head of the department Professor James Macleod had been on his summer holidays in Scotland while these experiments were carried out.

On his return Macleod took charge of the project begun by Banting. It was at his instigation that the next important event in the insulin story took place. Macleod suggested that Banting and Best discuss their experimental findings at the departmental journal club.

Meeting of University of Toronto Physiology Journal Club, November 14, 1921

This was the first time when Banting presented the results of experiments he had carried out in the Department of Physiology at Toronto University.

Journal clubs are an interesting educational institution. I have drawn some of this material from an excellent article published by Dr Mark Linzer in Postgraduate Medical Journal (1987) 63, 475–478.

The earliest reference to a journal club was by Sir James Paget, a British surgeon who referred to "a small room over a baker's shop near Saint Bartholomew's Hospital gate in London between 1835–1854 where some of the pupils, "making themselves into a kind of club,… could sit and read the journals and where some, in the evening, played cards." Sir James had noted that the library was small without a suitable reading room.

The Canadian physician William Osler had established a Journal Club in Montréal in 1875 to buy and distribute periodicals which he considered too expensive for purchase by an individual including himself. It is said that this form of informal gathering for purposes of study and discussion had probably arisen in Germany which in the second half of the 1800s was considered the leader in medical studies and training.

Journal Clubs in today's medical institutions are generally an informal in-house gathering of a group of medical graduates engaged in either research or hospital medical practice who discuss a particular topic. In research circles, an experimental project being carried out at the time is presented by those working on it. Other research workers as well as senior members of the staff including men and women, who may be involved more in patient care than actual laboratory research, also attend the meeting to hear the latest views or experimental findings on a particular subject.

After the presentation the subject is open for discussion by all attending. Often ideas from "the left-field" by senior men or women not directly involved with the project under discussion provide ideas for younger researchers who may not have been thinking along those lines.

This, in fact, was what happened to Banting and Best at their presentation to the Journal Club in the Department of Physiology at Toronto University on November 14, 1921.

The date of the presentation was of interest and importance to Frederick Banting who had wanted to present his first paper on insulin on his 30th birthday and was able to do so. According to a diary entry dated November 14, 1921, Banting had the ambition of writing one article every year for five years. He was also undecided as to whether he should pursue further studies for a fellowship of the Royal College of Surgeons or to continue with research in physiology. He still wanted to get married but it was unclear whether his feelings for Edith Roach had cooled in spite of her rejection. In part the diary entry read, "Only time alone I suppose will solve these problems. At present it behoves me to study and work at the internal secretion of the pancreas and if possible isolate it in a form that will be of use in treating diabetes."

As was the custom, the head of the department, Macleod chaired the meeting. Charles Best showed the charts and Banting did the talking.

During the discussion which followed one question and suggestion was particularly important and helpful for the researchers.

Norman Burke Taylor (1885–1972), a physiologist complimented the two researchers on their work, then asked if they had considered a longevity experiment using their insulin extract on one of the dogs.

No, Banting and Best had not thought of this. More surprising perhaps was that the head of the department, Macleod had not mentioned it to Banting either. Given Macleod's interest in diabetes and the fact that he had written a textbook on the subject, it was surprising that researching a potential treatment for a chronic condition, in this case diabetes, had not included a longevity experiment. After all, treatment with insulin was going to be needed long-term.

The following day, November 15, 1921 Banting and Best, with Macleod's agreement, made plans to start on the longevity experiment.

A problem which had frustrated the pursuit of insulin was the time-consuming exercise of obtaining an extract from the islets of Langerhans after tying off the pancreatic duct and waiting for the gland to breakdown, a process which was slow, and in the end yielded only a small amount of material from which to make the extract.

Banting had read about the work of Laguesse (1861-1927) mentioned earlier in this account. One of this French scientist's contributions was that the pancreas of newborn and foetal animals had plentiful islets whereas the mature pancreatic cells (acini) which produced the digestive juices developed largely after birth. This meant that foetal and newborn animals were a better source of insulin. In more recent times Laguesse's findings had been repeated and confirmed by the work of the physiologist Anton Carlson in Chicago in 1911.

So where could Banting get supplies of foetal pancreases? Memories of childhood came back to him. He had been brought up on a dairy–farm. Banting recalled his father's habit of breeding cattle just before slaughter to make them better feeders which increased their weight and therefore the price they commanded from meat-producing merchants.

Most of the abattoirs were situated in the north-west section of Toronto. Next day, early in the morning, the two fledgeling researchers went to the William Davies Company's abattoir. On the floor of the section where the animals were slaughtered various parts of the carcasses were rejected and left on the floor to be cleaned by young employees. Banting and Best found pieces of offal lying about on the cement floor in higgledy-piggledy fashion. Banting pointed out the "sweetbread" which included the pancreas removed from calf foetuses to Best.

An extract made from this material was injected into dog 27 which had had it's pancreas removed three days earlier. The blood sugar dropped promptly and within 24 hours it's urine was completely free of sugar.

Banting and Best clearly recognised the importance of this finding.

On November 23, 1921 Banting gave himself an injection of 1.5 cc of this extract. He suffered no ill-effects.

In all likelihood this was the first injection of insulin in a human being. The two types of injections of the extract, into the vein and under the skin, were used by Banting because they are the two commonest routes of injecting insulin into diabetics.

Both Banting and Best realised that only injections of the extract seemed to be effective in lowering glucose levels.

Unfortunately as had happened previously, the excitement and exultation of the two researchers over the results obtained with the foetal extract used in dog 27 was short lived. On the afternoon of December 2nd, barely a week after they had begun the trial, four hours after an injection, dog 27 had convulsions, lost consciousness for several hours, and died the next day.

Still Banting was nothing if not determined. He had seen that the extract had worked albeit only for a few days. Once again, he maintained, in fact stated emphatically, that the experiment demonstrated that the extract had been a success – it's just that the patient died.

So the challenge became one of getting both parts of the exercise to work, firstly the patient (the dog) surviving the extract and secondly, demonstrating that the extract reduced the level of blood glucose.

Marjorie (Dog 33), the Favourite

As suggested by Dr Norman Taylor during the discussion at the Journal Club meeting four days earlier, the two researchers began the longevity experiment.

On December 6, 1921 dog number 33, later to be called Marjorie, whose pancreas had been removed on November 18, became the subject of the second longevity experiment.

They used the extract prepared from the pancreases of unborn calves. The experiment continued through 70 days which was 10 times longer than any previous experiment. Much to the delight of the researchers Marjorie passed sugar free urine without any marked increase in blood glucose levels.

Banting's persistence was rewarded beyond all expectations. During her longevity experiment Marjorie had received more pancreatic extract than any other subject including humans. In total she had been controlled with daily injections of insulin extract for 70 days.

Unfortunately, published or unpublished records of Marjorie's condition are incomplete. However, a further test was carried out by Banting and Best between January 21 to January 23, 1922. They discontinued injecting Marjorie with the extract. The effect was dramatic. The dog became profoundly weak and was hardly able to stand, let alone walk. Upon resumption of the injections of extract on January 24 and 25, Marjorie showed clear improvement.

At the end of 70 days, Macleod had expressed doubt on the validity of the experiment questioning whether all her pancreas had been removed.

In order to resolve this matter Banting sacrificed Marjorie on 22 January 1922 and asked Dr William Robinson, an experienced pathologist, to perform a post-mortem examination. This confirmed that the dog did not have any significant amount of pancreatic tissue left.

The success of this experiment however, was marred by a weakness seen more than once in experiments carried out during the period of experiments on isolating insulin. This was poor record-keeping. Accurate and legible record keeping is of critical importance in scientific work especially when the notes are handwritten. More than once in the story the reader will come across this failing which was not restricted to Banting. However in this particular instance, namely the important experiments on Marjorie, poor record–keeping was to raise question marks on the validity of the experiment later.

There is no record of questions being raised by anyone including Macleod on this in the work carried out by Banting, Best or Collip. A more serious consequence of this lapse was to occur at a critical part of this account a little later.

The two other negatives of the experiment were firstly, abscess formation at the site of the injections which the researchers attributed to impurities in the extract and secondly, the need for the large quantity of extract needed to treat the hundreds of diabetics. Foetal calf pancreases only produced a small amount of extract from each batch.

Banting and Best, with a few changes in their methods of extraction, succeeded in making an extract from an adult pancreas. On December 11 one of the dogs was given the extract from its own pancreas (which had been removed to make it diabetic). There was a significant drop in its blood sugar level four hours after the injection.

Thus in a few weeks Banting and Best had progressed from the cumbersome and slow method of obtaining effective extract from ligating the pancreatic duct and waiting for weeks for the pancreas to shrivel before crushing the islets to the new method of obtaining supplies of extract from fresh whole pancreas. This method also removed the need to use the recently discovered method of using foetal glands.

The use of adult beef pancreas for producing insulin remained a major source of insulin for diabetic patients around the world for the next 40 years and continues to be used in many parts of the world to this day.

Enter the Wizard

"I experienced then and there all alone....the greatest thrill which has ever been given me to realise."

Collip on "seeing" insulin.
January 16, 1922.

As mentioned earlier there were two matters which troubled Banting during the early weeks of summer 1921. Firstly he believed that the poor conditions in the laboratory were the reason for the post-operative complications of infection in the experimental animals. This had been resolved with the assistance of Dr Starr who had made the necessary arrangements for Banting to perform the surgery in the far better facilities in the surgical premises of the hospital. This had happened before Macleod had returned from his holidays.

The second matter which troubled Banting was the variability in the effectiveness of the extracts being prepared by himself and Charles Best. At the beginning of the project while discussing it with Macleod Banting, on more than one occasion, had met a visiting biochemist who was in Toronto as part of a travelling fellowship awarded by the Rockefeller Foundation.

James Bertram Collip, a year younger than Banting, had gained an honours degree in physiology and biochemistry in 1912 followed by a PhD in biochemistry. He was known for his expertise in preparing extracts. Among his younger associates and students Collip was referred to as the "Wizard".

Upon hearing about the extract on which Banting and Best had been working, Collip had stated that within two weeks he could refine the extract and make their preparation more effective. Even though Macleod had previously not agreed to include Collip in the team, he now changed his mind.

The exact date of Collip starting on the project is not clear but most of the records indicate that it was around Christmas time in 1921. Collip himself recognised and acknowledged the work that had been done by Banting and Best before he had joined them. In a letter preserved in the University of Alberta archives, he had written to Dr Tory in Edmonton in January 1922 in which had said, "There are three of us associated with Prof. Macleod in this work. Dr Banting a surgeon and Mr Best a recent graduate first demonstrated the feasibility of use of pancreatic extract. I was invited to share in the future developments and definitely took over the chemical side as well as part of the physiological side of the problem."

Within weeks Collip had developed an effective extract. It will be recalled that Charles Best had noticed a difference in the effectiveness of the extract caused by changing the concentration of alcohol used in the process. With his experience Collip knew that further refinements of that particular step might prove successful.

He was right.

By patient experimentation Collip discovered the exact concentration of alcohol at which the solution consistently yielded insulin. Michael Bliss accessed a privately held undated, handwritten letter by Collip which dates the discovery on either January 16 or 17, 1922. Describing that moment many years later (1949), Collip wrote, "I experienced then and there all alone in the top story of the old Pathology Building perhaps the greatest thrill which has ever been given me to realise."

At a dinner given in Collip's honour in 1957, Dr R.F. Farquharson, Professor of Medicine at Toronto, speaking of that historic incident, quoted Walter Campbell, the physician at Toronto General at the time of the discovery who had said

"Collip then actually saw insulin."

The form of insulin developed by Collip was a white powder. Its further refinement some years later as described in this account would constitute one of the more dramatic chapters in the Insulin story. Even at the time of the discovery Collip had been unable to control his excitement. In a letter written in early January 1922 to H.M. Tory the president of the University of Alberta he provided further details saying:

"I will never regret having decided to spend a year near Professor Macleod. At the recent Conference at Yale he stood out most obviously as the leading man present. Last spring the old problem of diabetes was again taken up for re-investigation in his laboratory. During the summer such encouraging results were obtained by Dr Banting and Mr Best that in the fall the scope of the work was much enlarged. I was given the chemical side and a good part of the Physiological to push along with.

I planned a series of experiments the results of which when obtained gave me a direct lead to the solution of the basic functional derangement in diabetes. The crucial experiment was tried out just before the Christmas break and the results were so striking that even the most sceptical I think would be convinced. I have never had such an absolutely satisfactory experience before, namely going in a logical way from point to point into an unexplored field building absolutely solid structure all the way. However to make a long story short we have obtained from the pancreas of animals a mysterious something which when injected into totally diabetic dogs completely removes all the cardinal symptoms of the disease. Just at the moment it is my problem to isolate in a form suitable for human administration the principle which has such wondrous powers, the existence of which many have suspected but no one has hitherto proved.

If the substance works on the human it will be a great boon to medicine, but even if it does not work out a milestone has at least been added to the field of carbohydrate metabolism. Professor Graham was in my laboratory today discussing the whole matter and in the course of a few days time we hope to have had a clinical test made. If it works we will turn over in all probability the formula to the Connaught Anti-toxin laboratories for manufacturing purposes.

To be associated in an intimate way with the solution of a problem which for years has resisted all efforts was something I had never anticipated. I only wish that the various papers which will be published on this work were coming from Alberta rather than Toronto."

Like many researchers, Collip had limited knowledge outside his field. A humorous incident at the time of his starting on the insulin project revealed that he had had little experience in studies on diabetes. A few days after starting on isolating an extract, Collip came to Banting and Best, saying that he was not able to obtain any insulin from his extract. Further inquiries revealed that the laboratory assistant Collip had sent to the butcher for "sweetbread" had brought him specimens of liver and thymus but not the pancreas! Collip who had clearly handled the material had not realised that the pancreas was missing for the simple reason that he did not know what a pancreas looked like.

Charles Best, the student had a field day! He related the incident, with embellishments of his own and certainly with relish, to anyone who would listen.

It didn't take long for the story to get back to Collip. He was not amused and never forgave Best.

The reader would not fail to realise that looking at the entire team involved in the original discovery of insulin only Banting had any practical experience starting with his familiarity with foetal and adult pancreases because of his upbringing on a dairy farm whereas the head of the department where the work was carried out namely James Macleod had little if any experience in working with large animals. Neither did he have any experience in treating diabetics because he had gone from graduation to physiology research.

As the incident above illustrates Collip although possessing a Doctorate (PhD.) in biochemistry had never actually seen, let alone handled, a pancreas.

Then there was Best who was a student with book knowledge of diabetes as understood by his lecturer and through the information contained in the textbook written by the same man.

Yet as history would show, all three of the team felt that they had played important roles in the discovery of insulin. And all three wanted to share the spoils of victory. Little wonder that the story has retained a fascination for many.

A later letter to Tori from Collip spoke of his success in isolating an effective extract.

"Last Thursday, January 19, (1922) I finally understood the method of isolating the internal secretion of the pancreas in a fairly pure and seemingly stable form suitable for human administration. It was tried out on one case in the clinic with such encouraging results that today $5000 has been placed at our disposal to secure apparatus, four assistants etc to rush the work for the next four months in the hope that we may establish a block of clinical evidence which will prove either the value or the worthlessness of this substance in treating diabetes in the human."

Many years later (1949) Collip recalled that momentous experience saying, "I experienced then in there all alone in the top story of the old pathology building perhaps the greatest thrill which has ever been given me to realise."

What Collip was referring to as a "pure and stable form" was actually insulin which he had managed to isolate as a powder. Giving the details of this at a medical dinner in honour of Collip in 1957, the then Professor of Medicine at Toronto University, Dr R.F. Farquharson quoted Walter Campbell as saying, "Collip then actually saw insulin."

Although the white powder produced by Collip was later found to have many impurities it was a vast improvement on the previous efforts of Charles Best.

The potency of the extract was confirmed by its desired effect on rabbits. Unlike previous preparations the new extract was not followed by abscesses at the site of the injections.

Collip's extract was ready for trials on human diabetics.

While Collip had been busy refining the extract, an incident involving Banting is perhaps more of interest than importance in the insulin story.

Banting's Secret – and Unauthorized Trial of Insulin
What are friends for ?

Between December 12 and December 16, 1921 Banting and Best used the extract they had prepared from whole pancreases of dogs and cows on one of their dogs. The results of the test were inconsistent but at least some blood sugar levels fell spectacularly. Banting seized upon this "success" to charge headlong to the next stage.

He gave himself an injection of the extract in the skin without any ill-effects. He told Best that he had decided to test the extract on a human without telling anyone. Strictly speaking, they should at least have spoken to James Macleod or Banting could have sought the views or advice of his mentor and guide, Clarence Starr.

The use of untested and untried medications or "cures" on human beings was not as highly regulated then as it is today. However such activities were frowned upon certainly by members of the medical and pharmaceutical fraternity. The historical records of the highly regarded Lilly Company show that the original founder dealt only with doctors in medical practice and did not sell his products to anyone else. Neither did he permit his chemists to produce any patent medicines.

Whether Banting was aware of these opinions and practices relating to untried medications is unclear but given his bull-at-the-gate approach, it is unlikely he would have been held back by any such opinions or advice.

He telephoned one of his classmates from medical school.

Joe Gilchrist had graduated from Toronto University medical school in December 1916. Shortly afterwards he had developed diabetes. Following a restricted diet prescribed by Francis Allen of New York, he was managing fairly well except for the weight loss which always accompanied such a diet.

In October 1921, after an attack of influenza, Gilchrist's condition became much worse.

Therefore when his classmate Fred Banting phoned on December 20, Gilchrist was willing to try anything to halt the deterioration in his condition.

There are few details of this incident except the brief remarks on an index card contained in the Banting papers:

"December 20, phoned Joe Gilchrist.
  – Gave him extract that we knew to be potent – by mouth –
empty stomach.
  December 21 – no beneficial result."

Clearly a fundamental fact of human physiology that the acid in the stomach will have destroyed the the extract had escaped both Banting and – the physiology student – Best.

One can only speculate on Banting's decision to expose Gilchrist to the risks inherent in injecting an untried substance into a human subject based on inconsistent results obtained in animal experiments. It was only good fortune which averted a major, even fatal, disaster. This attitude of Banting which verges on the cavalier, was an area which should have been picked up by his supervisor namely Macleod who appears to have been largely "missing in action" perhaps as much from Banting's pigheadedness as from his (Macleod's) disinterest and indifference.

Gilchrist maintained a friendship and professional relationship with Banting and later worked with him in the Veterans' clinic which had been established to provide Banting with an official position and facilities to treat diabetics.

The Toronto University archives preserve a document which lists the physicians "prominent in treating diabetes," meeting in Toronto in the early months of the release of insulin. Together with well-known names including senior physicians from America such as Robert Williams and Elliott Joslin is included the name of Joe Gilchrist next to Banting's.

Whatever his faults, and he had many, Fred Banting placed great emphasis and reliance on friendship as he did with Gentleman's agreements which he habitually sealed with a handshake.

The First International Presentation by Banting 20th December, 1920

"I became almost paralysed."

Frederick Banting.

"The importance of the reports lay not in the form but the substance."

Henry Macleod Best.

Six weeks after the Journal Club presentation, the Toronto team Banting, Best and Macleod travelled to Yale University in New Haven, Connecticut to present their findings at the meeting of the prestigious American Physiological Society on December 30, 1921.

It was well known that Banting was nervous when it came to public speaking. This had been evident even during the presentation to the much smaller group at the Journal Club a few weeks earlier. Therefore he was glad to have Charles Best showing the charts and sharing the stage with him.

Of the three, only Macleod was a member of the Physiological Society. The others in the team were there by invitation.

It is unclear whether Banting had known that, in addition to the physiologists, several well-known American physicians had also been invited to the meeting because of their interest and experience in diabetes in children and adults. So in addition to addressing physiologists with far greater experience in laboratory research than he had, Banting was also going to face men recognised for their expertise and experience in the treatment of diabetes in children and adults. Many of these men, in addition to their clinical experience in treating diabetes had, over the years, also engaged in laboratory experiments on diabetic animals. Therefore in both fields, namely laboratory experience and treatment of human diabetics in adults and children, Banting was not in the same league as the physicians to whom he was going to present his experimental findings.

The physicians in the group included Elliott Joslin from Boston, Rollin Woodyatt from Chicago, Anton Carlson from the Mayo Clinic and Francis Allen from New York.

One of the attendees who would play a critical role later in the story was J.H.A. Clowse, originally a research chemist but at the time the research director of the pharmaceutical company Eli Lilly of Indianapolis. Banting need not have feared the experienced older men. Without exception they were courteous and patient with the two presenters as they were towards the members of the Society which had opened its doors to them when it need not have. Usually only members attended its meetings but given the topic of the presentation the Society had invited the physicians.

The one man in the audience who was well known to Banting through his writings was Francis Allen. It was Allen's operating technique for removing the pancreas from dogs which Banting had used on his own experiments.

Allen's knowledge of the effects of diabetes on human beings as well as in animals was extraordinary. Many regarded him as the foremost American authority on the subject and referred to him as "Dr. Diabetes".

He is remembered for his intensive research carried out over a period of three years during a fellowship at Harvard University medical school between 1909 and 1912.

Allen had operated on hundreds of dogs, cats, guinea pigs and other smaller animals. Certainly in the United States there was no one in his league as far as experimental work on diabetes was concerned. An unfortunate drawback for Allen was his rather dour personality and, in the opinion of patients, their relatives, and also some attending nurses, his insistence on a strictly restricted diet at times combined with exercise as the treatment for diabetes which led to his patients becoming markedly underweight, often emaciated.

What is often omitted when this criticism is levelled at Allen is that the restricted diet was all that was available as treatment at that time. Following such a diet often turned patients into extremely thin, haggard, "just skin and bone" individuals which alarmed their relatives as well as members of the staff.

Before insulin there was no other treatment for such patients.

On the other hand, Allen was known amongst his younger colleagues as an extremely patient, humble and friendly teacher.

During his fellowship at Harvard he had produced a publication, *Studies Concerning Glycosuria and Diabetes.*

Although Allen himself had referred to the work as "an enlarged journal article", it was actually a book of some 1100 pages and contained a bibliography of over 1200 references. It was not accepted by any of the journals of the day and was later published as a book, *Glycosuria and Diabetes* by W.M. Leonard of Boston and released for sale by Harvard University Press of Cambridge Massachusetts early in 1913. The expenses had been subsidised by Allen's father.

To say that Banting was nervous would be an understatement. His own recollection was recorded in one of his personal papers.

"When I was called upon to present our work I became almost paralysed. I could not remember, nor could I think. I had never spoken to an audience of this kind before – I was overawed. I did not present it well."

The meeting was chaired by Macleod. This was common practice as the presentation was from his department. Also, he was the only one of the presenting team who was a member of the Society of Physiologists.

Except for Macleod, Banting didn't know any of the members of the Society, nor any of the invited guests. He had little if any experience in engaging in a group discussion.

I could not find any information on Banting's preparation for this meeting. Normally there is a considerable amount of rehearsing and question-and-answer sessions in the days or weeks before the actual presentation. Usually a senior member in the department, even the Head of the department who in this case was the only member of the presentation team who was a member of the Society helped in preparing the individual who was going to present the material.

The obvious person to help the team was Macleod. He was, as the head of the department, familiar with the work which was to be presented and which he claimed, had been done under his "direction". Macleod, an experienced researcher was also known for his prowess in public speaking. Being a member of the Society he would no doubt have been familiar with the kind of questions to expect from the members.

Did he knowingly throw Banting to the wolves?

Stories of the strained relationship between Macleod and Banting are repeated frequently in both the books on the discovery insulin.

After Banting's presentation Macleod invited questions from the audience.

The response was immediate.

Several hands shot up. In fact several members were on their feet, ready with questions. This was, after all, a meeting to discuss the results of research being carried out in Toronto. Such meetings were usually a "no–holds–barred" session and common courtesies were often ignored.

Banting quickly found himself in hot water.

"You say you are conducting longevity experiments but your data show that the experiments on your dog number 33 have not even been completed."

"Well, yes but dog 33 is the second one on whom the experiment is being performed," stammered Banting and immediately regretted his answer realising too late that what he thought was a killer blow was yet to come.

"Yes." The unnamed physiologist paused and looked around before delivering the knockout punch.

"But didn't you say that the first dog died?" Another look at the audience before turning away without waiting for an answer—he didn't have to.

Banting heard someone in the front row mutter, "the experiment was a success except that the patient died."

Several questions were directed at the measurements of various chemical components in the blood which had not been presented by Banting for he had concentrated primarily on removing the pancreas to make the dogs diabetic, then used the pancreas to make an extract to be injected into the animals.

His omissions had been quickly detected by experienced researchers who lost no time before attacking him in the very areas where they could see he was vulnerable. Clearly flustered, Banting continued to utter mumbled incoherent replies. No mercy was shown by physiologists to the practising physician. "How dare he invade our turf ?" may well have been the thought underlying the attack on the inexperienced visitor.

Macleod, himself a physiologist, came to Banting's rescue but only after the nervous researcher had been thoroughly humiliated.

If the presentation at the Journal Club in his own backyard in Toronto had been, for Banting, akin to a being placed in a crucible, the experience in Yale was like being subjected to the fierce flames of a blow torch.

Given his experience and background it is reasonable to question Macleod's contribution or rather the lack of it in this aspect of research which he had authorised and with which he was supposedly familiar. There is no doubt that he will have known the kind of questions Banting was likely to face in New Haven but there is no record of Macleod helping Banting in his preparation for the presentation. Certainly on the basis of the information available Banting was quite unprepared for the onslaught by men far more experienced in the field of experimental physiology. Macleod would have known this but had done nothing to prepare Banting or his own student Charles Best for this.

One particular incident can be described to illustrate how out of their depth the two Torontonians were on that day in New Haven.

One of the invited physicians to the meeting was Anton Carlson who had worked with pancreatised dogs. Commenting on the death of dogs in Toronto after Banting's operations, Carlson said that some of his dogs had lived much longer than Banting's. This was perhaps Carlson's way of drawing Banting's attention to the causes of death in laboratory animals and giving him an opening to describe some of the difficulties in the kind of research he was carrying out. Unfortunately Charles Best did not grasp the hint and interjected that Carlson may not have removed all of the pancreas in his dogs!

What Best did not know was that he was speaking to a man some 25 years older who was the Chairman of the Department of Physiology of the University of Chicago and a world authority on several aspects of physiology including the digestion of starches (carbohydrates). Carlson had written a book on "the control of hunger in health and disease" in 1916. He had been involved in experiments with animals for many years. Fortunately the experienced researcher and departmental chairman took the student's remark in good humour, responding with "young man, you might be right!"

Best never forgot this incident nor Carlson's gracious handling of his impertinence.

In short, the initial public presentation was at best a learning experience for Banting and Best and at worst a serious lapse on the part of Macleod.

Banting was devastated and never forgot the humiliation. Nearly 20 years later he recalled that he had not slept a wink on the train that night. In fact he had not even gone to his berth but had sat up in the smoking compartment silently cursing Macleod as an impostor and himself as a nincompoop. He decided that he had to learn to write clearly, legibly, precisely, explicitly and then be able to talk convincingly, freely and unhesitatingly.

He felt he knew Macleod for what he was, a talker and a writer. In Banting's opinion, "apart from his pen and his tongue, Macleod would not even be a lab man for he had no original ideas, and no skill with his hands in an experiment.

He only knew what he read or was told and then he could rewrite or retell it as though he were a scientist and a discoverer. It was foolish to spend weeks and months working night and day at experiments and then have them told beautifully by someone else who had the art as though they were his ideas and his works."

Reactions to Banting's Presentations
A Medical Grapevine.

Both of the first two meetings during which Banting's and Best's work was discussed, namely the Journal Club on November 14, 1921 and the meeting in New Haven on friday afternoon December 30, 1921, had far-reaching consequences which may not have been appreciated at the time. The reason for this is possibly because the information was passed informally by word–of–mouth through what some may choose to call a medical grapevine.

Dramatis Personae:
 Llewellis Franklin Barker, a physician from Johns Hopkins.
 Hospital, Baltimore.
 Elliott Joslin, the diabetes specialist from Boston.
 George Clowse, Senior Executive and Research Director,
 Lilly Company.
 James Macleod, Professor of Physiology, Toronto University.

Settings:
 A suite in a hotel in New Haven, Connecticut.

A Function room in a hotel in Arkansas.

The Library of the Department of Physiology Toronto University.

The first piece of information to spread through the grapevine from the presentation at the Journal Club in the library of the Department of Physiology on the afternoon of November 14, 1921 was by a physician who after the meeting had engaged Banting in conversation. Banting and Best were collecting their charts and slides. They did not know the man who approached them and assumed that he was a visitor.

Llewellis Franklin Barker (1867–1943) had graduated in medicine from Toronto University in 1890. After his internship he had gone to Johns Hopkins in 1892 to work in William Osler's clinic. However he had remained in touch with his alma mater through regular visits to Toronto University. He never returned to work in Toronto but remained at Johns Hopkins where he succeeded Osler in 1905.

After a brief conversation with Banting and congratulating him on the "exciting findings" Barker left the meeting and shortly afterwards returned to Baltimore.

A week later he went to a meeting of the Southern Medical Association in Arkansas. This was a very conservative group of physicians who dated the beginning of their organisation from the early 1900s, the first meeting documented as having been held in 1906. Also at this meeting was the well known diabetes specialist from Boston called Elliott Joslin who had been invited to present a paper on a recently discovered "cure for diabetes" called insulin.

Barker like most, if not all, members of the Association was familiar with the name of the Boston physician and his reputation and interest in the study and medical care of patients with diabetes. They had met during Joslin's visits to Baltimore for the meetings of the Osler Club of which Joslin was a foundation member. The high regard in which Joslin was held by the members of this austere organisation was evident in a remark by Dr. James S. McLester, who when introducing the guest speaker, said "to paraphrase a well-known advertisement, when we think of diabetes we think Joslin."

What Barker told Joslin about the research in Toronto and the findings presented by Banting and Best at the Journal Club meeting was entirely new to the Boston physician.

As was typical of him, Joslin lost no time in putting pen to paper.

In a letter to Macleod dated November 19, 1921 Joslin asked the professor if the work in his department had been published or was about to be published anywhere.

"Naturally if there is a grain of hopefulness in these experiments, which I can give to patients or even can say to them that you are working upon the subject, it would afford much comfort, not only to them, but to me as well, because I see so many pathetic cases."

According to the records in the book by Bliss, Macleod was unusually prompt in his reply to Joslin which was dated November 21, 1921.

"It is true that we have been doing work on the influence of pancreatic extracts, which has yielded most encouraging results," Macleod answered, "but I would rather hesitate to attempt the application of these results in the treatment of human diabetes until we are absolutely certain of them. Dr Banting and Mr Best who have been doing this work, are to report their findings at the meeting of the Physiological Society at New Haven, by which time we expect to be in a position to come to a definite conclusion. I may say privately that I believe we have something that may be of real value in the treatment of diabetes and that we are hurrying along the experiments as quickly as possible."

There is no record of Macleod ever saying to Banting or Best that he believed that what the two researchers were doing could be of "real value in the treatment of diabetes." Neither did he say anything to this effect when introducing Banting or when commenting on Banting's presentation at the New Haven meeting. The possibility of the clinical value of the extract which Banting was presenting to the group of physiologists, none of whom would have had any experience in treating diabetes, might have lessened their thirst for Banting's blood in New Haven. But Macleod had kept silent as Banting was being put to the sword.

Joslin's own impressions of the New Haven meeting were recorded in an interview with the military and medical historian William R. Feasby many years later.

"Dr Banting spoke haltingly, but we could gather that really something had happened and that the sugar in the blood of the dog had dropped. It was a little difficult to catch the whole story, but later this was emphasised and beautifully told by Dr Macleod. There was little praise or congratulation, and a moderate amount of friendly but serious criticism of the work.

The physiologists present deeply resented the interest and enthusiasm of us clinicians who were there and evidently hinted that never again would we be invited to come to the meeting."

Once again Joslin's comments reveal the difference between those engaged in the practice of medicine namely "clinicians" and research workers such as the physiologists in the Society at New Haven where Banting's paper was presented.

The very fact that the blood sugar of the dog had dropped was seized upon by the practising physicians like Joslin who had longed for this to occur in his patients. Never mind the design of the experiment and the stringent requirements of laboratory methods and experiments. All the practising physician wanted was for the suffering child or adult to be spared the consequences of a high blood sugar. If there was something, call it what you will – a potion, or an extract or whatever, if that's what it was going to take to lower the blood sugar, physicians who at that time could only watch as literally hundreds of diabetics were barely surviving on a starvation diet, would have been prepared to seize upon any solution which promised a lowering of the blood sugar. For them the effect of Banting's extract on that one dog was cause for unbridled enthusiasm, optimism and hope.

Remember that hope was what had been denied to the patient throughout the history of this condition which had brought untold suffering to man for literally thousands of years.

George Henry Alexander Clowse, the Insulin Missionary

"..that insulin missionary, G. H. A. Clowse, who has ceaselessly wandered up and down the length and breadth of this land, untiring in his endeavour to be useful to all."
Elliott P. Joslin, in the preface of *Treatment of Diabetes Mellitus*, third edition 1923.

Of even greater importance to the insulin story especially in advancing the development of the hormone and making it suitable for use in diabetes is one other person to whom Barker had spoken about the work in Toronto.

His name was George Clowse, the Research Director of Eli Lilly Company of Indianapolis, Indiana.

Clowse, who had a reputation for cultivating friendly relations with physicians especially the Heads of clinics and departments, made a note to attend the New Haven meeting. This was going to have far-reaching consequences which remain relevant to this day and could not have been apparent to any of these men at the time.

When Macleod returned to his hotel room in New Haven after the meeting he received a phone call from Clowse. Whether or not Macleod knew that Clowse, in addition to his position at Lilly was in his own right a respected medical researcher is unknown but he would have guessed that the man on the end of the phone did have knowledge beyond that of a pharmaceutical representative especially when Clowse unhesitatingly expressed the unsolicited opinion that the evidence presented by the two researchers was "convincing". Then, ever the entrepreneur, Clowse asked the Professor whether the Eli Lilly Company could collaborate with his researchers in preparing the extract for commercial distribution. Macleod's response was guarded to say the least or the less charitable might say, negative. Macleod, as he had said to others stated that the work was not sufficiently advanced for commercial preparation but that Clowse's suggestion would be "borne in mind."

Many years later Clowse said, "It is true that Banting presented his material somewhat haltingly and certainly very modestly. However, anyone who was at all cognisant with the subject must have realised that a great discovery had been made and that provided the work could be brought to fruition there was every prospect that an important means of treating diabetes would be developed."

This forthright assessment of the work in spite of all its shortcomings showed the sharp intellect of the researcher in Clowse. His subsequent offer of collaboration for large-scale production of Insulin showed his appreciation of the importance of translating laboratory discoveries into practical solutions – in this case, making insulin available for the treatment of diabetes.

He would no doubt have noticed Banting's plight when fielding the questions from the physiologists. Was his comment regarding anyone being "at all cognisant with the subject" a veiled criticism of the way the many physiologists, with little if any experience in treating diabetes, had engaged in belittling Banting. Was this done to see if Macleod, who had chaired the meeting and could have helped Banting, would react ? He didn't.

Yes, there would be money in it for the Lilly Company but more importantly, here was an opportunity to relieve the suffering of millions who had suffered since time immemorial.

Much is made of the importance and value of "communications" today but "the grapevine" remains as popular and widespread as a means of disseminating information as it appears to have been 100 years ago.

Another physician who had recognised the potential of the work being done in Toronto was Frederick Allen who wrote to Macleod a few weeks after the New Haven meeting.

"I hope your work with the pancreas extract is progressing satisfactorily. With the beginning of our animal experimentation here, I shall probably go ahead with plans I have had for a long time, in the direction of an extract. Our methods are totally different from yours. You would not only have priority, but, if you have solved the initial difficulties, your method is better than mine could ever be. I've merely thought of my method as a means of escaping those difficulties, and it may have some value for other purposes at least, so I should probably give it a try. It is high time we had some treatment beyond mere diet, though I recognise the difficulties in the way of a practical application of any extract."

This passage is included because it demonstrates several qualities in Allen's character. He was humble when referring to his own knowledge and experience. He did not mention his own writings and experiments when giving unstinting praise and encouragement to the young investigators in Toronto. How different this was from their treatment by the physiologists. Allen's comment on the need for "some treatment beyond mere diet" highlights the priority clinicians like Allen gave to finding a more effective method of treating their patients.

This essential difference between practising physicians and laboratory/research workers is often missed especially in books written for the lay public. It may also explain at least in part, the delay in bringing the results of research to those suffering from diabetes. This in fact did occur in the case of insulin when it was introduced in Britain.

The mixed reception given to the New Haven presentation and other early papers written by Banting and Best was, in my opinion, placed in proper perspective by Charles Best's son Henry Best who observed that "…the importance of the reports lay not in the form but the substance".

This was the voice of a senior academic. Best had served as President of Laurentian University. He was also a mature observer – 66 years old – at the time of the publication of his book.

He said, "In succeeding years, there have been harsh criticisms of the weaknesses in the early papers. Flaws there were, certainly, but the result was of world – shaking importance, and that is what mattered. The lack of experience of Banting and Best, the initially poor working conditions and lack of financial and other support make that achievement all the more impressive."

Henry Best did not engage in trenchant criticism especially of Macleod and the treatment he meted to both Banting and Best especially Banting but one could read a wealth of meaning when he speaks of the lack of "other support".

The First Trial of insulin January 11, 1922

Banting barred by a Bureaucrat

Repeatedly seen in the story of the earlier and critical stages of the experiments which led to the discovery of insulin is the one difference between Banting and the other members of the team. Only Banting was a practising physician, in medical jargon, a clinician.

The others were teachers and researchers who were not involved in the care of patients.

Macleod, although a medical graduate, had spent his life as a physiologist and worked as a researcher and teacher. Best was still a student. Collip who joined the other three was, like Macleod, a researcher and lecturer at the University of Alberta.

This difference between Banting and the other three is significant. It explains Banting's focus, some may say preoccupation, throughout the quest for insulin and which continued with added vigour following its discovery.

Therefore it is not surprising that as soon as the extract was found to work in a dog, Banting could not wait to try it on a human patient.

He had never forgotten the fateful event which he had recorded in his notebook at 2 am on October 31, 1920.

Of the entire team Banting alone had never lost sight of what he considered to be the central and overriding issue of the work which had occupied – and driven – him over the preceding 12 months. He had never lost sight of the fact that the critical test of the entire exercise would be the effect of the extract on a human patient. And the thought uppermost in his mind and heart was to be part of the team carrying out this 1st "clinical trial."

Today's medical researcher may, on the one hand cringe at such audacity but on the other, secretly envy Banting's freedom to even contemplate testing a product of research on a patient so soon after its discovery.

Today's scientist trying a new treatment developed in the laboratory has to jump through several hoops of medical bureaucracy including the agreement/approval of the head of the relevant department (like Macleod in this story), and ethics committees. If the project is approved, the researcher/s organise clinical trials on a large number of individuals often in several hospitals, at times in different countries. This can take months, even years, before a product developed in the laboratory can reach a patient suffering from the condition for which the new treatment has been developed.

Another reason for delay is hesitation on the part of practising physicians to expose their patients to a previously untried treatment. A treatment effective in an animal does not guarantee that it would produce the same result in a human patient.

"Never be the first or the last to try a new treatment" was an oft-repeated maxim of one of my teachers during my years of medical training.

Therefore it was no surprise that Frederick Banting met with firm, and vocal, resistance from the practising physicians of Toronto General Hospital when he approached them to try his extract on one of their patients.

In addition to the reasons described above, the personalities of senior physicians and surgeons, who were often older and more experienced than the researchers also played an important part in deciding whether Banting's experiment was going to be permitted on human subjects. Although some may have been at least willing to listen, others flatly refused to allow their patients to be used as guinea pigs.

It is part of history that Banting's priorities meant little to others. It was Banting who pushed and pushed hard to test the extract on a human patient. I could not find any evidence in the literature of any other members of the original, or the later expanded team, pursuing a clinical trial as a priority. This is not surprising given the fact that, as stated previously, only Banting had been a practising physician.

The first and most formidable obstacle in Banting's way was the physician in charge of the Department of Medicine at Toronto University.

Duncan Archibald Graham (1882–1974) had the reputation of holding "the first position in the British Empire of Chair of Clinical Medicine at the University of Toronto" in 1919.

At Toronto General Hospital he was the head of the Department of Medicine and Physician–in–Chief. Although his postgraduate studies had mostly been in pathology, his position at the hospital was mainly administrative. He insisted on patients being admitted to wards where they were treated by physicians with the training appropriate for treating that particular ailment.

Described by his biographers Robert B. Kerr and Douglas Waugh as dour and ruthless, Graham gave Banting short shrift. He flatly refused to appoint him to any position in the hospital. He stated bluntly that Banting was a surgeon who had not been in medical practice for more than a year. Neither did he have any formal qualifications to experiment on patients. He dismissed the persistent outsider with a double-barrelled retort.

"What right have you to treat diabetics?" followed by

"How many of them have you ever treated?"

It was well known that Graham was friendly with his fellow Scotsman Macleod. The relationship between Macleod and Banting had been uneasy including at least one confrontation.

Had Banting's limited clinical experience and background been related to Graham by the physiologist?

Whatever the information he had on him, Graham made it clear to Banting that he would not to be allowed anywhere near a patient in hospital. If Graham thought that he had put the impertinent outsider in his place he had underestimated the opponent.

The dour Scotsman's stubbornness was matched by Banting's refusal to take no for an answer. Switching his point of attack, Banting turned to Macleod and pestered him relentlessly.

Eventually one Scotsman managed to persuade the other.

Graham agreed – but with one stipulation. The extract was to be injected in a patient in the appropriate medical ward at the direction of the physician in charge. The physicians in charge of the medical wards at that time were Drs. Walter Campbell and Almon Fletcher.

Graham still would not budge on Banting. He was not allowed to enter the ward, or even to witness the injection been given.

An ironic twist which further embittered Banting was that while he and Best were outside the ward, the first injection of *their* insulin extract inside the ward was making history.

Banting's version of the event as recorded in his 1940 memoir is quoted in the book by Michael Bliss as follows :

"We went to the hospital and remained in the corridor and a houseman injected it into the patient. We had advised Campbell concerning the time for taking samples of blood for blood sugar estimations and also concerning specimens of urine. We waited around for the first specimens and could hardly contain our suppressed excitement.

This was in reality the first human diabetic to be treated.

When the specimen of urine arrived we were told that it would be tested in due course. We asked for a small sample, just a few drops, but we found the whole sample was the property of the hospital, that all specimens would be done together along with samples of blood and that we would be given the results on the following day. There was a cool atmosphere about the place but there did not seem to be anything to do so we went back to the laboratory."

In other words, there was no special treatment for what to Banting was a unique medical event of historical significance.

The two researchers, thoroughly deflated by the intransigent medical bureaucrat, returned to the laboratory. Clearly the medical administrator's priorities were different but what is surprising is its acceptance by Banting given his "short fuse."

Could the insulin hero be mellowing?

Success Denied Success Achieved

January 11, 1922

On January 11, 1922 in Ward H of Toronto General Hospital, a resident medical officer by the name of Ed Jeffrey injected the extract prepared by Banting and Best in two divided doses of 7.5 mls. into each buttock of a 14-year-old boy called Leonard Thompson.

The two researchers had tried the same extract on a dog, then on each other before giving an amount from the same batch to the hospital.

Leonard Thompson, a 14-year-old whose diabetes had been diagnosed in 1919 had been a patient of the hospital for two years. He had been treated by dietary restrictions. At the time of the discovery of insulin Thompson's condition had deteriorated and he was mostly "skin and bone." As was common, the appearance of such patients was never forgotten by those who saw them in that state. In this particular case the boy's father had brought his son to the office of Duncan Graham. Graham's secretary at the time, Stella Clutton never quite recovered from the shock of seeing the child. When interviewed by Michael Bliss for his book some 60 years after the event, she told Bliss that she had never seen anyone alive who was as thin as that boy. She said that his appearance reminded her of "victims of famine or concentration camps."

Banting, still smarting from having been barred from being present and part of the history–making first injection of an effective extract in a human subject was dealt two more sickening blows. The fall in blood sugar and the resulting reduction in the amount of glucose in the urine was, to put it mildly, disappointing. To make matters worse, an abscess developed at the injection sites.

There was a terse and damning response from the physicians.

"No clinical benefit was observed, the experiment had been a failure.

No further injections were to be given."

So it had all come to nothing.

Or, had it?

Remarkably even though he was disappointed, Banting remained doggedly determined.

There was an interesting detail associated with this hospital experience. Many years after the event it was discovered that the clinical notes in the records of Leonard Thompson's first failed experiment the extract had been referred to as "Macleod's serum."

Given that Duncan Graham had been the one to reject Banting's request, could Macleod have exaggerated his own role in the preparation of the extract to overcome Graham's objections and at the same time get the pesky Fred Banting off his back?

At this point we return to the work of Collip who had produced an extract the biochemist believed was suitable for human trial.

THE FIRST SUCCESSFUL INJECTION OF INSULIN IN A HUMAN PATIENT JANUARY 22, 1922

At 11 am on Monday, January 22, 1922 Leonard Thompson was injected with five mls of the new extract which had been prepared by Collip.

The patient tolerated the extract without any complications. He was given a further 20 mls at 5 pm followed by two injections each of 10 mls the next day.

Within 24 hours, the sugar had disappeared from the urine and the level of blood sugar had dropped five-fold.

Even more remarkable was the effect of the injections on the patient himself which was obvious to all.

"The boy became brighter, more active, looked better and said he felt stronger."

This was a quotation from a paper written by Banting, Best, Collip and the hospital duo of Campbell and Fletcher. The fact that the last two were physicians who came on the scene only at the time of giving injections and had no role whatsoever in the research which led to the discovery of insulin may confuse some readers but the inclusion of the names of all involved in a particular exercise including the clinical application of research findings as happened here is common practice.

Although not recognised as such at the time but perhaps a portent of things to come, there was no extract on the 25th and 26th of January because Collip had run out of supplies and was making a new batch.

As he had done with Banting, Duncan Graham did not permit Collip to witness Thompson's treatment because – wait for it – Collip was "not a doctor and did not hold an appointment at the hospital."

What is intriguing is the absence of Professor Macleod throughout these dramatic events. Was he still holding firm on his stated view as reported, on the project "going up in smoke" and his opinion as stated in the book he had written on diabetes that there was no single factor within the pancreas to influence the level of glucose in the blood ?

At this point further progress in the the discovery and development of insulin was overtaken by a force beyond the control of the scientists, professors and even the Titans of hospital administration. It was the press.

THE POWER OF THE PRESS.

Given Macleod's hesitation, even fear, of premature publicity of the discovery it was not surprising that he tried to discourage newspaper reporting at that time. As events unfolded he was to be reminded of something that many men and women in academia have experienced but have often struggled to accept, namely the power of the press.

The Toronto Star

The Toronto Star, the first newspaper to report the discovery of insulin was at that time the city's leading newspaper. It had surpassed the sales of its competitors several years earlier in 1913. The newspaper owed its rise to a dynamic young journalist, Joseph Atkinson who, in December 1899 at the age of 32, was appointed editor.

Atkinson, like many printers of the past, wanted the paper to be for ordinary people. He himself had been one of eight children brought up by his widowed mother who took in boarders to support her family. After his mother died Joe left school at the age of 14 to work in a woollen mill to support the family. Unfortunately the building was destroyed by fire shortly after he joined and he then had to rely on charity for food. Atkinson never forgot this. Largely self-taught through extensive reading, he was convinced that liberalism was the best way to improve the lot of the common man. Under his stewardship the paper grew in quality and circulation. By 1917 its price had risen from one cent to two cents per copy.

From 1920, employing the latest printing technologies, the Star had become a leader in newsprint innovation.

At the time of the discovery of insulin in 1922 the Star had also acquired its own radio station giving it a decided advantage in publicising the epoch-making event.

The reporter to break the insulin story was a young man called Ross Greenaway. The sequence of events began with a familiar incident.

Banting, during a bout of heavy drinking, was talking to one of his former teachers, Dr G. W. "Billy"Ross, who ran a medical practice in Toronto.

This was after Collip had taken over the production of the extract and Duncan Graham had excluded Banting from the hospital. Banting was considering withdrawing from the entire insulin project but Best had managed to persuade him to stay the course.

Ross, who had always liked Banting, often used to meet up with him and, in all likelihood, had been told by Banting of the first injection of the extract given to a patient in Toronto General Hospital on January 22. Ross Greenaway was one of Ross's patients.

The young reporter had somehow discovered the name of the patient. He promptly contacted Leonard's father who confirmed the story. Greenaway lost no time in going to the Toronto University's Physiology Department and barged into Macleod's office.

As he had done with all previous inquiries including the earlier ones from Joslin and G.H.A. Clowse, the professor tried his hardest to discourage the young reporter's expectations. This time however he was not talking to medical men but a young and enthusiastic newsman. Greenaway would not be denied. Promising Macleod that he would take care to emphasise that the investigation was, to use Macleod's expression, "only at a preliminary stage" so as not to build false hopes, he lost little time in running to his editor.

I found online a cutting from the Canadian Press Dispatch dated January 10, 1922 stating,

"Progress is reported to have been made in an experiment attempting to find a cure for diabetes which Professor John Macleod has been conducting at the Toronto University Laboratory for several months.

It was only a day or two ago that the first injection of the extract was given to a human being. This is a boy of 13 in the Toronto General Hospital. So acute is diabetes in young people that very often hope of recovery is in vain. It was as a last resort that permission was granted to the Toronto research men to experiment with this boy. So encouraging was the first treatment, that it has been announced that these treatments will be continued every day."

The reader will not have failed to notice the discrepancy in the dates of the first successful trial with the extract. The first with Banting and Best's extract on January 11 had failed. Some of the dates in various reports are inaccurate.

If Banting, when talking to Billy Ross was drunk it is likely that he was confusing the disastrous first attempt on January 11 with the successful second lot of injections given to Thompson on January 22. It is also possible that Banting wanted it documented that the first injection of insulin in a human being was from an extract prepared by him and his assistant Charles Best.

Little has been written about the importance of this newspaper report in giving impetus to efforts to further refining of the extract so that it could be safely employed in the treatment of diabetes. From this point on there was marked acceleration on several fronts which culminated in the refined preparation reaching the level of safety which satisfied all involved that the discovery could be reported. The report which took place in May 1922 will come a little later.

I discussed the issue of preliminary (? premature) reporting of events such as this with Vijendra Kumar, the retired editor of one of the more influential newspapers of the South Pacific region, The Fiji Times. The much-admired editor was held in esteem by the entire multiracial community of the region as much for his integrity as for his fearless pursuit of truth. Though retired, Vijendra is still very much in touch with current affairs and regularly reads several international and local newspapers.

I asked him if Greenaway should have waited until the May 1922 report to the American Association of Physicians meeting in Washington.

He seemed surprised by my question. His view was that the information Greenway had would have been rightly considered "of worldwide interest and there was no hope of him letting go. His editor would have impressed on him the importance of keeping his ear to the ground right through to the end," said Vijendra Kumar.

(Another reporter employed by the Toronto Star at that time was Ernest Hemingway. It is said that at the time Hemingway was also writing the novel *A Farewell to Arms*. He was living in a residential hotel in downtown Toronto. The hotel was owned by the same Gooderham family who had donated the land for building the Connaught Antitoxin Laboratories which, in 1922, produced the first supplies of insulin.)

A comprehensive coverage of the discovery appeared in the Toronto Star on Wednesday, March 22, 1922.

The front page which I found online, featured under the title of the newspaper, its 30th year of production, the copy consisting of 28 pages, dated Wednesday, March 22, 1922, 5 o'clock edition and its price, two cents.

"Toronto Doctors On Track Of Diabetes Cure" screamed the front page headline. A group photograph of Banting, Best, Collip and Macleod was captioned, "Have They Robbed Diabetes of Its Terrors?"

The most significant statement in the journal article according to The Star was, "the effects observed in the pancreatised animal have been paralleled in man."

When Greenaway asked when the treatment would be available, Banting replied, "not for 3 to 6 months."

The Star continued its coverage the following day under the headline

"Diabetes Work Epoch-Making Say Physicians."

The main source of Greenway's articles was Banting. One of the subheadings of the front page feature was

"Banting Stakes His All On The Result."

The Star, the leading newspaper in Toronto at the time remained at the forefront of reporting on developments in the production of insulin and later, on the critical role played by the Eli Lilly Company. Greenaway did not contribute as many articles after this initial period.

The News Heard Round the World.

"One of the greatest achievements of modern medicine."

The formal announcement of the discovery of insulin was made on May 3, 1922 at a medical conference in Washington DC.

During April the findings were carefully summarised in the form of a paper to be submitted for presentation at the meeting of the Association of American Physicians scheduled to be held in Washington on May 3rd, 1922.

The authors of the paper, "The Effect Produced on Diabetes by Extracts of Pancreas" were listed as Banting, Best, Collip, Campbell, Fletcher, Macleod and E.C.Noble.

It was agreed that, for the first time, the term "insulin" be used to replace the earlier term "Isletin" which had been used by Banting and Best.

Unlike the robust discussion which had followed Banting's presentation in New Haven in December 1921, this paper delivered by Macleod was met with approval and excitement. It was given during the noon-hour session.

Other presenters at the meeting had been asked to keep their papers short in order to give the Toronto presentation pride of place.

One of the physicians, Dr S. Solis – Cohen said, "this study, so careful and comprehensive, this work so thorough in its execution and so clear in it's presentation, may justly be called epoch making. I'm glad that I have been privileged to hear the paper."

Francis Allen, respected and widely regarded as a leading diabetologist in the world, agreed.

"If as seems to be the case, the Toronto workers have the internal secretion of the pancreas fairly free from the toxic material, they hold unquestionable priority for one of the greatest achievements of modern medicine, and no one has a right to divide the credit with them," he declared.

Rollin Woodyatt stated that he was convinced that the Torontonians had successfully isolated the elusive pancreatic extract.

"I think this work marks the beginning of a new phase in the study and treatment of diabetes. It would be difficult to overestimate the ultimate significance of such a step."

Woodyatt moved that the Association tender a standing vote of appreciation.

Elliott Joslin, the respected Boston physician also regarded as one of the world's leading specialists in diabetes was present at the meeting. Commenting on the standing ovation by the usually staid and conservative physicians, Joslin said that in his 20 years with the association – he had been a founding member – he had never seen such a demonstration of emotion. He also said that it was the first time any presentation had been honoured with a standing ovation.

It is of historical interest that neither Banting nor Best was present at the meeting. Each claimed that the expenses for the trip were beyond their means. This was unlikely as both of them at that time were on a salary. Furthermore, had they really needed financial assistance to go to Washington, one phone call to Clowes at the Lilly Company would have in all likelihood received the required financial assistance.

In the normal course of events questions following the presentation would have been directed at the two workers who had made the discovery. There was no mention of their absence during or after the presentation which, as already noted, was made by the Head of the Department, James Macleod. Perhaps the difficult interpersonal relationships within the group which had become common gossip on the medical grapevine was the root cause of Banting and Best being absent.

The importance of the discovery was clearly recognised by all present at the meeting.

It also bears repeating that from the first steps taken on this journey by Banting on May 17th, 1921, less than 52 weeks had elapsed before the discovery of insulin was announced that day in Washington.

Walter Campbell (1891–1981) who was present in Washington at the time of the presentation was in no doubt about the importance of the occasion. Toronto General Hospital's Senior Physician never forgot the occasion. As late as 1962, 50 years after the event, he said, "We had it made."

Banting's and Best's absence from the meeting in Washington is part of the historical record.

Perhaps these two young men, in spite of their age, knew that history also has a memory.

A Postscript

It is interesting that there is no mention of the Washington meeting in the book by Henry Best. We can speculate on the reasons for this. Did Charles Best not write about this because he and Banting did not go to the Washington meeting? Given the careful cataloguing of Charles Best's scientific writing why was this not included in the family records especially as he and Banting were the two leading authors of the paper which was read at the American Association of Physiologists meeting?

A historian may be forgiven for not giving this particular presentation the importance given by physicians.

Of course the explanation could be as simple as the material escaping the attention of Henry Best given the very large amount of material contained in the collection which he and his helpers had to sift through when deciding on what was to be included and what was to be left out of his book.

Scientists engaged in medical research today may view wistfully Banting's and Best's 12–month journey from the beginning to the end of the discovery of insulin. The various requirements which have to be satisfied before today's researchers are permitted to start a project like this one would require them to work their way through many checks and balances about which I have spoken in another part of this account.

The Summer of 1922

The Purification and Development of Insulin

"Until insulin circulates in diabetic veins"
Frederick Banting March 31, 1922.

Some may argue that the proven effectiveness of an extract containing the "internal secretion"had successfully completed the critical part of Banting's research. After Leonard Thompson several other patients were treated in Campbell's and Fletcher's clinic at Toronto General Hospital. They included Banting's friend Joe Gilchrist.

However, as has been previously noted, Banting never lost sight of the priority of pursuing Insulin as treatment for diabetes, and at no stage, did he lose sight of his ultimate goal.

Therefore, after the isolation of the extract, work continued with the aim of producing insulin in larger quantities.

A test of the potency of insulin in order to standardise the amount injected was worked out in which "one rabbit dose" was defined as the amount of insulin needed to lower the blood sugar level of a normal rabbit by 50%.

During February Banting and Best wrote papers for medical journals and also presented their findings to local medical bodies such as the Toronto Academy of medicine. Towards the end of February they had sufficient experimental evidence to support their claim that the extract was effective in treating diabetes.

They submitted an article to the *Canadian Medical Association Journal* which published it in its March issue. The authors of the article were listed in order as Banting, Best, Collip, Campbell and Fletcher. The paper also documented, for the first time, Collip's role in the development of insulin stating that "as the result obtained by Banting and Best led us to expect that a potent extract suitable for administration to the human subjects could be prepared, one of us J.B.C. (Collip's initials) took up the problem of the isolation of the active principle of the gland. As a result of this latter investigation, an extract has been prepared from the whole gland, which is sterile and highly potent, and which can be administered subcutaneously to the human subject. The preparation of such an extract made it possible to study its effects on patients with diabetes, the preliminary results of which study are herein reported.....

These results taken together have been such as to leave no doubt that in these extracts we have a therapeutic measure of unquestionable value in the treatment of certain phases of the disease in man."

The scientific value of this paper was dwarfed by the public interest generated by articles in newspapers. The intense public interest in articles published by prominent newspapers led by the Toronto Star understandably attracted far wider public interest than an article in a medical journal especially one like the Canadian Medical Association Journal which had a limited circulation within the small local medical fraternity.

Banting's Gentleman's Agreement with Collip

By early 1922 interpersonal rivalries and conflicts between the different members of the team namely Macleod versus Banting and Macleod plus Collip versus Banting plus Best had been resolved sufficiently for the team to work together. This was a gentleman's agreement sealed with a handshake by Banting with Collip and Macleod.

During the month of February and March 1922, plans for large scale manufacture of insulin in Toronto were well advanced. The earlier problems with purification which had been a major obstacle to its use in patients who had been treated with the extract prepared by Banting and Best had been resolved by Collip's contribution which had begun the week before Christmas 1921.

As noted earlier following the successful demonstration by the second injection given to Thompson the extract was being used in other patients in the hospital..

The Connaught Antitoxin Laboratories had installed new machinery in order to increase production of the extract. There was clearly an acute awareness of the plight of thousands of patients not only in Toronto but around the world who were desperately in need of insulin. Then, disaster.

"A Very Strange Mishap"

Collip, for reasons unclear, found that he could no longer make insulin.

Explanations for this totally unexpected lapse range from a deliberate act on the part of Collip to frustrate Banting to patenting the formula in his own name for financial gain, and to taking his expertise to another centre for adding to his academic achievements.

Just how a man with Collip's qualifications, obtained after years of training, could suddenly forget how to make the extract and not keep accurate records beggars belief.

Both the failure and the poor (? absent) documentation are problematic.

Bliss attributes Collip's failure to technical problems which were the bane of the manufacturing process in its early stages.

There has been very little discussion on this particular incident by any of the men involved. Even before he joined the team, Collip had commented that he would be able to produce an extract fit for human use in about two weeks. This was not surprising given his established reputation for expertise in this particular field. In addition to a Master's degree in chemistry (1913) and a Doctorate in biochemistry in 1916, Collip had an established reputation in the very specific field of making extracts. Given his comment on the short time of two weeks he needed to solve the problem raises the possibility that he had already guessed what the problems were which had proved a stumbling block for the inexperienced researchers. That he managed to produce the extract promptly would also suggest that he was right in his "diagnosis" of the problem.

"A very strange mishap" was how Henry Best described the sudden cessation of production.

Very strange indeed, for several reasons.

First of all, Collip was known for his conscientiousness in research and enjoyed a reputation as an expert in the field. Even if he was not able to put his finger on the problem immediately one would be right in assuming that he would know how to proceed. Yet he claimed that he had no explanation for his failure and expressed no intention to resolve the impasse. Particularly disappointing especially for Banting would have been the absence of any remorse or concern for patients with diabetes whose hopes had been raised by the recent discovery.

Even more puzzling is the fact that Collip left Toronto and returned to Edmonton (where he had accepted the position of Chair of the Department of Biochemistry) without giving any indication of wanting to solve the problem he was leaving behind for the other members of the team. This would be remarkable for any man in his position and reputation in this field.

So much for Collip's gentleman's agreement with Banting!

According to the University of Toronto records, Collip resigned. However in the Best family papers a letter dated May 10, 1922 from Charles Best to his father stated that Collip had been "kicked out."

This was one of the few matters in which Henry Best expressed reservations on the version of events presented by Michael Bliss.

In his book *Margaret and Charlie* Henry Best wrote:

"A doctoral thesis on Collip by Alison Li, written in 1993 under the direction of Professor Michael Bliss at the University of Toronto, adds considerably to our knowledge and understanding of Collip the man, and his career. However, despite her thesis director's later emphasis on the importance of Collip's contribution, this thesis of 289 pages has only ten and half pages on the discovery of insulin. Li's account skims over what happened in Toronto in late 1921 and early 1922: "for a period of several months that spring (1922), Collip was faced with the bleak fact that he had lost the ability to make potent extract. The cause of this problem is difficult to ascertain, but variations in vacuum pressure, temperature, and distilling time can wreak havoc on the preparation of biologic products. Also Collip's haphazard way of note taking did nothing to help."

Henry Best did not dwell on this but it is clear that he was less than satisfied with the version of events as presented by Bliss. Nor did he comment on Li's reference to the technical aspects of insulin production such as variations in vacuum pressure etc which would have been outside the field of the candidate's interest and expertise and which almost certainly came from Bliss's own information on the technical aspects of the production of the extract which he had acquired from discussions with chemists involved in the production of insulin as part of his own research in preparation for the book on the discovery of insulin he had written in 1982.

Henry Best went on to say that the details of the exact method used by Collip for large-scale production of the extract remained unknown. Some of Collip's recommendations for small-scale purification were used by Best and his colleagues later when during an intensive six-week period starting in mid-May 1922 they succeeded in modifying it for large-scale production. Since Collip did not leave Toronto till June 1922 he may well have assisted Best in his last weeks in Toronto but there is no record of this.

Given Best's comments in later years which emphasised his own role, at times without acknowledging the contribution of others, in producing insulin for large-scale use one might question whether the omission of Collip's contribution between May and June 1922 was conveniently forgotten.

Just as puzzling in "the Collip incident" was Macleod's explanation that Collip's extract "suddenly stopped working." So the Head of the department which had from the beginning adopted or, according to Banting at least, appropriated a supervisory and leadership role in the work, saw nothing unusual in Collip's lapse?

This was not the first time the question of Macleod's claims on the extent of his involvement in the work on insulin might raise eyebrows.

Collip's friendship with Macleod was noted by Bliss. Henry Best went further. He commented that in his textbook *Carbohydrate Metabolism and Insulin* Macleod gave Collip's method and indeed his entire contribution to the project "great prominence."

Macleod's high opinion of Collip was not shared by other men including the University of Toronto President Sir Robert Falconer and Dr.H. M.Tory, the President of the University of Alberta. Tory had no illusions about Collip's loyalties and said,

"I always believed that he was doing the manoeuvering himself, not anyone else. He has a fatal gift of interpreting a hint as an offer for the simple reason that he cannot see things outside their relation to himself."

Later a patent on insulin production was taken out to prevent commercial interests disadvantaging diabetics.

The Collip incident continues to fuel speculation and conspiracy theories to this day.

Banting's Gentleman's Agreement with Best

"If you get out, I get out."

Best to Banting, March 1921.

As a result of Collip's unforeseen – and unexplained – lapse there was a marked reduction in, then a total lack of, insulin for patients. This situation continued for several weeks. Leonard

Thompson who had remained in hospital because he had been doing so well while being treated with insulin, had to be discharged without any supplies. Predictably, his condition deteriorated quickly. We will return to his story later.

At this stage Macleod had taken over the running of the work on insulin. He appointed himself the leader of the team working on physiology. Collip was put in charge of biochemistry and the clinical/hospital roles were assigned to the physicians Walter Campbell and Graham. Aways the diplomat, Macleod added his fellow-Scotsman Duncan Graham to the medical team to work with Campbell. The inclusion of Graham may raise questions given that his official role was an administrative one. Was Macleod returning the favour to Graham for agreeing to Banting's first clinical trial of the insulin extract on Leonard Thompson?

Banting was assigned to carry out surgical procedures although there was little to do in that regard by this stage in the development of insulin. Best, like Banting, was not given any specific role. He knew that he had to write a thesis for his Masters degree. The subject for this as suggested by Macleod was "The Role of Pancreatic Extracts in the Utilisation of Carbohydrates by Diabetic Animals."

Banting, feeling that he was being bypassed by Macleod was incandescent with rage. Henry Best quoted a piece from one of Banting's unpublished manuscripts :

"None of them wanted anything to do with me.... During the latter part of February and the whole of March, I almost ceased to work. The whole affair was too much for my nervous system. The only means by which I could get to sleep was by taking alcohol. I do not think there was one night during the month of March 1922 when I went to bed sober.

About 10.30 on the night of March 31, Best came to my room at 34 Granville. It was blue with smoke.....

Best sized up the situation and proceeded to give me a setting out. He told me that Macleod was vexed because he was not getting extract with which to work. Collip was unable to make an extract as he had not written down his procedure so was unable to repeat it. Campbell was held up entirely.

Fitzgerald had offered to advance $5,000 for the provision of a laboratory in the basement of the medical building if we would commence work again".

I told Best I was not interested, that I would finish the teaching term with Henderson and then look for a place where there were decent people to live with.

Then Best said possibly the only thing that would have changed my attitude,

"What will happen to me?"

"Your friend Macleod will look after you," I said.

Best replied, "if you get out I get out."

"Here was loyalty.

I emptied my glass.

That is the last drink which I will ever take until insulin circulates in diabetic veins.

Shake on it Charlie.

We start tomorrow morning where we left off."

Over the next four to six weeks Banting and Best spent long hours, often 24 hours a day working on developing an effective extract in order to treat diabetes.

During this period the assistance and support provided by Clowse to the young investigators was of critical importance. Clowse's own experience and knowledge in large-scale production of drugs in which he had been engaged in the Lilly laboratories over many years was invaluable for Banting and Best. As will be seen later the success at this stage of Banting and Best's research in producing an improved extract owed much to the assistance provided by the experienced Clowse. Indeed when Best in January 1923 was appointed to head the production of the extract at Connaught Laboratories he and his team soon found themselves in trouble and once again had to be rescued by Clowse's team from Lilly.

As was typical of Banting he gave fulsome praise to Best for his hard work but also for his companionship and reliability.

Quoting from Banting's writings, Henry Best wrote:

"Best was pleased. We sat down and as we had done hundreds of times, planned experiments. For the succeeding months it was back to the old hard grind. Best and I worked in the sub–basement of the old medical building day and night. Time, meals, sleep, all were a secondary consideration. We had to get insulin into a form that was refined enough for continued clinical use. The atmosphere was different. We were happy. To Best must be given the greatest amount of credit for this phase of the development. It was he more than anyone else who bridged the gap between the test tube and the beaker and later, the large–scale production."

Banting made no mention of the fact that Best had made at least nine trips to Indianapolis in the summer of 1922 in order to seek assistance from Clowse and his colleagues.

Thus the second stage in the insulin story namely, the development of insulin, came to an end in the summer of 1922.

In retrospect, one could question the value of Collip's contribution which, as far as the development of insulin was concerned, amounted to demonstrating that further refinement of the original extract developed by Banting and Best was effective.

After his failure to continue with the project Collip left Toronto and it was Best who completed the development process for large–scale production of insulin at the Connaught Laboratories in the summer of 1922.

Thus for Charles Best the fortuitous summer holiday-job turned into a life–changing event.

As stated previously, the subject of the thesis assigned by Macleod, was directly related to the work being done by Banting and Best. The subject for this was suggested by Macleod. It was "The Role of Pancreatic Extracts in the Utilisation of Carbohydrates by Diabetic Animals."

The thesis was due on 1 May, 1922.

Had Banting walked away at this stage Best's thesis would have been in jeopardy. Given Banting's intoxicated state it is unlikely that Best's plight would have crossed the older researcher's mind.

Little wonder that Best was concerned about the possibility of Banting giving up on the insulin project as related above. He would have been relieved to have succeeded in getting the volatile, hot-tempered senior member of the team to change his mind.

According to Henry Best the preparation for Charles Best's Master's thesis took place "amid the confusion and frenzied activity of the winter and spring of 1922. He was so busy with the preparation of scientific papers on the discovery of Insulin and the practical challenges of large–scale production that he had little time to spend on the thesis. He stated at one point that he had written the text the night before it was due."

One bound copy of Best's thesis was filed in the department and another with the University of Toronto.

An intriguing fact emerged when many years later, in 1975, Linda Mahon, the younger sister of Charles Best's wife Margaret Mahon, wanted to find a copy of the thesis because there has been a query arising from London (from whom was not stated) asking for the date of publication and the title. Neither the departmental records nor the university library had the thesis entered in their files. Each source listed it as "missing."

As for gentleman's agreements on which Banting always placed great emphasis, it appears that Best had respected Banting's commitment while Collip had not. As will be seen, Banting kept his side of the bargain and shared most of his rewards with Best. It took him a long time to forgive Collip, which he eventually did.

So When Was Insulin Actually Discovered?

Henry Best, after examining the family papers in preparation for writing his book was confident of the date of the discovery.

He stated that "certainly by December 1921 Banting and Best believed that they had discovered Insulin."

He quoted the letter written by Best's fiancé's younger sister Emma who was 16 at that time. She wrote to an uncle, Bruce Macleod.

"Charlie is not going home this Christmas but he and a Dr. Banting with whom he was doing research work all summer, are going to speak before the American Medical Society by invitation. I tell you what, old Dear, they are stirring up a lot of excitement in the city. They have completed a cure for diebeaties (*sic*). Just now they're trying to get the stuff so it can be drunken. They have it so that they can put it under the skin but that is sort of painful so they're trying to see how it can be taken by mouth. Imagine those two. One twenty two and the other twenty nine. Dr Banting was the one who set my leg for me."

(Banting who had been in general practice had also done a term of orthopaedics during his training.)

This part of Henry Best's book also mentioned, and not for the first time, that Best's fiancé Margaret Mahon, according to her entries in the family papers "helped write part of the paper presented at the Journal club in Toronto and the one to the physiology society at Yale as well as a published piece in the medical journal afterwards."

This is contained in the letter by Margaret Mahon to the same uncle, Bruce Macleod to whom her younger sister had written earlier. She said, "If you would care to see it I will send you a copy of the first paper when it appears in the medical journal. Charlie wrote the paper ably assisted by your niece. He dictated parts to me and I have developed a real interest in diabetes."

Unfortunately there are few details on Margaret's assistance other than typing Charles Best's notes or dictation. This entry in the book was just before the presentation to the American Physiological Society at Yale University in New Haven on 30 December 1921.

Henry Best concluded this section in his book with the following observation,

"In succeeding years, there have been harsh criticisms of the weaknesses in the early papers. Flaws there were, certainly, but the result was of world –shaking importance and that is what mattered. The lack of experience of Banting and Best, the initially poor working conditions and lack of financial and other support, make their achievement all the more impressive."

This was one of the few occasions on which Henry Best expressed an opinion and it sounds like the voice of a man of considerable authority and experience which of course he was. At the time of the publication of his book Henry Best was 63 years old. He had been the President of Laurentian University and was a respected historian.

It is interesting that he did not express an opinion on a subject emphasised repeatedly not only by Michael Bliss in his book but also, especially in his later years by Charles Best, namely the part played by James Macleod throughout the story of the pursuit of insulin.

PART THREE
INSULIN EUPHORIA

Insulin a Triumph of Hope

I trace the rainbow through the rain
And feel the promise is not vain,
That morn shall tearless be.
George Matheson (1842-1906).

STORIES OF JOYOUS RELIEF

The First Patients to Receive Insulin

The most important effect of insulin on the lives of those who suffered and those who tried to care for the suffering can be described in a single word. Hope.

Insulin saved lives. It changed lives.

The number of lives saved starting from its discovery in 1921 now numbers in the millions.

Before Insulin there was no hope because there was no treatment. If a child developed diabetes his or her lifespan could be measured in months. A minor infection rapidly progressed to accumulation of acid in the blood (acidosis) and death in a matter of hours. Hardly ever did a young person afflicted with the condition survive for more than 2 to 3 years.

A starvation diet which only brought at most, a few years provided the patient did not develop an infection which was usually the forerunner of the fatal train of events described above.

Throughout my forty years in a consultant practice dominated by diabetes I never ceased to be amazed by the changes brought about by the use of insulin especially in children and young people.

But first, by way of contrast, let us remind ourselves of the plight of those who lived with diabetes before the discovery of insulin.

Born Before Insulin

The story of young Frances Putnam

"Shush, never mention the word diabetes."

Frances Cabot Putnam, born in 1897, came from the upper echelons of Boston society. She was the daughter of Dr. James Jackson Putnam, a pioneer neurologist and professor at Harvard Medical School. Her story was described in her mother's memoir.

During one of her frequent trips to Europe for holidays, Frances at age 15, developed the classical complaints of diabetes namely excessive thirst, weight loss and tiredness.

The family memoir does not mention the word diabetes. In polite society, in common with other diseases, afflictions remained anonymous.

She was treated with dietary restriction but within 12 months, having lost more weight, was becoming increasingly tired. Her condition was described by her mother in the family memoir as, "one day with Baby (the family's name for her) was enough to make me realise that she was losing ground."

The doctors could not offer Frances or her family any help other than rest and dietary restriction as treatment for her condition. Even more tragic was the fact that before insulin doctors could not even offer what every person and their families yearn for– hope.

Donald M. Barnett in his book Elliott P. Joslin, MD: A Centennial Portrait described the final days of the 15-year-old:

"On a cold rainy evening, when Frances' parents returned from dining with the Emersons (Ralph Waldo Emerson's son) of Concord, Massachusetts, Mrs. Putnam was "struck by Baby's extreme paleness, but she was in good spirits and put on one of her dancing-school dresses because she thought (a guest) would like to see it."

From that point on, her mother wrote in typical stoic fashion, "Frances grew steadily worse until Friday, December 12, 1913, when she fell asleep soon after midnight and died peacefully about 8 o'clock."

So near …. The tragedy of Paula Inge

If one heartbreaking story can be more tragic than another, the story of Paula Inge, the 11-year-old daughter of the Dean of Saint Paul's Cathedral, W. R. Inge may be recounted.

When she developed diabetes in November 1921, Paula's condition was so severe that the doctors predicted death within a month. However showing a maturity beyond her age she followed her diet religiously and was still alive 12 months later. Although insulin, at least in Toronto, had been available since November 1922, when Paula's father sought information on its availability in England he was told by Henry Dale that the treatment was in the experimental stage and not available. He was only half right. Insulin was in the experimental stage but it was available and had been in use for treating patients in Toronto since mid-1922.

Some historians blame the cautious approach adopted by British authorities at the time for the delay in using insulin there. In Britain in the winter of 1922–23 less than 50 patients in eight different hospitals received insulin. Tragically, Paula Inge was not one of them.

Yearnings of the Desperate

"The full beseeching of 100 pairs of eyes"

In my opinion the most moving description of the hopes of patients is found in the recollections of a nurse who worked with Frederick Allen at his hospital in Morristown in 1922.

Speaking of "the mere illusion of new hope" cajoling patient after patient into new life she said,

"Diabetics who had not been out of bed for weeks began to trail weakly about, clinging to walls and furniture. Big stomachs, skin-and-bone necks, skull-like faces, feeble movements, all ages, both sexes – they look like an old Flemish painter's depiction of a resurrection after famine. It was a resurrection, a crawling stirring, as of some vague spring time."

Then recalling the atmosphere and the reaction of the patients on hearing that Dr. Allen had come back she wrote:

"Bed immediately after dinner was the rule for our patients. But not that evening. My office opened on the big centre hallways. I could see them drifting in, silent as the bloated ghosts they looked like. Even to look at one another would have painfully betrayed some of the intolerable hope that had brought them. So they just sat and waited, eyes on the ground.

It was growing dark outside. Nobody had yet seen Dr Allen. His first appearance would be at his dinner, which followed the patients' dinner hour. We all heard his step coming along the covered walk, past the entrance to the main hallways. His wife was with him, her quick tapping pace making a queer rhythm with his. The patients' silence concentrated on that sound. When he appeared through the open doorway, he caught the full beseeching of a hundred pairs of eyes. It stopped him dead. Even now I am sure it was minutes before he spoke to them, his voice curiously mingling concern for his patients with an excitement that he tried his best not to betray.

"I think," he said, "I think we have something for you."

The Drama of Salvation

"Probably no one thing in medicine has ever stirred the physicians in the United States as much as the development of this pancreatic extract."

Francis G. Benedict.

The transformative effect of insulin defied description. No superlative was adequate for the experience and emotions felt by the afflicted who experienced it and by the parents, relatives, and friends who witnessed it. The doctors who had treated patients with diabetes were speechless with wonder – and relief.

Those with religious convictions ascribed the discovery of insulin to divine intervention just as many in the past had believed diabetes and other conditions to be a punishment visited upon human beings by angry gods.

Of the physicians in the English-speaking world arguably the most articulate was the Boston physician Elliott Proctor Joslin (1869–1962). A Harvard professor who had written the first English language textbook on diabetes in 1916, Joslin at the time of the discovery had seen in excess of 1000 patients with the condition. Young people who developed diabetes before the discovery of insulin usually died within 2 to 3 years. Joslin, a pious, ascetic Puritan who was known to carry a copy of the New Testament in his coat pocket (but never quoted it to his patients) unhesitatingly likened the remarkable changes he witnessed in the treated patients to the resurrection and salvation of the dead and the suffering as recorded in the book of Ezekiel in the bible.

"Prophesy unto the wind, prophesy, Son of Man, and say to the wind, Thus saith the Lord God: Come from the four winds, Oh breath, and breathe upon these slain, that they may live.

So I prophesied as he commanded me, and the breath came into them, and they lived, and stood up upon their feet, an exceeding great army."

Similarly, Michael Bliss who had tried to remain objective and had done so with admirable restraint throughout his narrative could not help being moved by the accounts of the effect of insulin on patients. Like Joslin had done years before him, Bliss also described the discovery in biblical terms including the resurrection. The opening paragraph of his book read as follows,

"The discovery of insulin at the University of Toronto in 1921–22 was one of the most dramatic events in the history of the treatment of disease. Insulin's impact was so sensational because of the incredible effect it had on diabetic patients. Those who watched the first starved, sometimes comatose, diabetics receive insulin and return to life saw one of the genuine miracles of modern medicine. They were present at the closest approach to resurrection of the body that our secular society can achieve, and at the discovery of what has become the elixir of life for millions of human beings around the world."

At the conclusion of his work Bliss once again waxed biblical and wrote,

"With insulin, the stone was rolled away, and diabetes became a matter of life, not death."

Even many years after the discovery of insulin the reaction of my patients on starting insulin after suffering from the effects of diabetes almost defied description. I came to understand why men like Elliott Joslin who saw numerous examples of the effect of insulin on their patients used biblical analogies.

The commonest response of the physicians who actually saw insulin-treated patients whom they had treated before insulin was quite simply, utter speechlessness. Elizabeth Hughes, whose story is recounted below and who had never met Joslin until he came to see her in Toronto following her rescue by Banting's insulin injections, described the Boston Brahmin as, "simply adorable" and "the sweetest man who just stood there looking, smiling and not saying anything."

For Joslin to be lost for words, the occasion had to be special.

The New Haven meeting had, for the first time, permitted the invited group of physicians mainly from the United States to glimpse the possibility of possible relief for the suffering diabetic. Descriptions of the severely affected, especially children and young adults, with daily and ever-present reminders of a uniformly fatal condition appeared in every description of the malady. No one recovered from diabetes. The only treatment offered was a severe reduction in food intake which often led to a worsening of the physical condition even if it afforded some relief from thirst and the loss of sugar in the urine. The host of suffering children and young adults and their families leapt at the slightest hint of treatment – any treatment.

The next largest group of individuals involved in the care of patients afflicted with diabetes were the physicians. Information on the medical grapevine after the Journal Club meeting has been described earlier. The results of the trials on humans reported at the Washington meeting on May 3, 1922 were seen as the most dramatic announcement in the history of diabetes in its thousand year history.

Every physician at the meeting who had himself cared for a patient with diabetes or knew of a diabetic patient realised that at last there was something which had until then been but a forlorn hope. Never mind the pros and cons of the design of the experiment and the hesitant even bumbling presentation by the inexperienced Banting. All that had struck them like a flash of lightning was the reduction in blood glucose when the dog had been given the extract of insulin.

The effect of the announcement on all who heard it was predictable, understandable and inevitable.

There was a veritable stampede for insulin, for Toronto, for Banting.

Every contact with any promise of access to the "magic potion" was worth pursuing. Requests to the Toronto researchers by Allen paled in comparison with the rush of concerned physicians, friends, and relatives and parents of diabetic children. Every avenue was used in the hope of obtaining insulin. Business contacts, fellow workers and even, as related in another story, golf buddies, were asked to plead for help. That diabetes was a fatal condition was well known and therefore such desperation for a possible cure, yes cure, was understandable even though doctors including Banting had repeatedly emphasised that insulin was a treatment but not a cure for those who suffered from diabetes.

Here are a few examples of the changes in the lives of several young men and women who had lived through a period before the discovery of insulin and then were treated with it. The changes experienced by them as well as their families and the medical and nursing staff who looked after them are best described in some of the case histories of that period.

Banting's First American Patient

Banting's first American patient was Elizabeth Hughes, the daughter of prominent American Jurist and politician Charles Evans Hughes Sr. (1862–1948). Hughes had been widely tipped to win the 1920 presidential election against Warren G. Harding but was beaten narrowly. Harding had persuaded the highly regarded Hughes to accept the position of Secretary of State. Earlier in his career Hughes had become close friends with Associate Justice Oliver Wendell Holmes Jr, the son of the prominent Boston physician Oliver Wendell Holmes.

Even though she was only 11 at the time she was extremely articulate and her account is one of the most frequently quoted. At the time of Elizabeth's birth in 1907 her father was the Governor of New York having defeated the newspaper tycoon William Randolph Hirst in the 1906 gubernatorial race.

In 1918 Elizabeth developed the classic complaints of diabetes with unquenchable thirst, alarming weight loss, the predictable onset of lack of energy followed by profound weakness. At that time sufficient was known about the condition to know that there was no cure and in the case of children death was inevitable usually within 2 to 5 years.

She was taken to Francis Allen, the best known diabetes doctor in New York. Allen confirmed the diagnosis of diabetes and put Elizabeth on a daily diet of 400-600 Calories and total fasting one day a week. This made Elizabeth less thirsty but reduced her weight to an alarming 55 pounds (25 kilograms). A nurse experienced in the treatment of diabetes who had been trained at the clinic of Boston's Elliott Joslin, was employed to help in the child's treatment.

Allen had been present at Banting's presentation at Yale in mid 1921. As soon as the discovery of insulin was announced on

May 3rd, 1922, Allen was inundated by phone calls from anxious parents of diabetic children.

In the case of Elizabeth Hughes, it was her mother Antoinette Hughes who used the direct approach and addressed her letter personally to Frederick Banting pleading for help for her "beautiful but depleted and reduced daughter". She received an answer by return post.

On August 15, 1922 Elizabeth Hughes became Frederick Banting's first American patient.

Elizabeth Hughes recovered and lived to the age of 74 years. She had led a full life, married and had three children. She had kept her diabetes a secret from all except her husband who was told a week after they had become engaged.

BANTING'S HOUSE CALL TO GIVE INSULIN TO THE FIRST PATIENT IN AMERICA

James Dexter Havens (1900-1960)

This 15-year-old developed diabetes in 1915 and was treated by Dr. John R. Williams, one of the leading physicians in Rochester, New York. He was treated with a restriction diet which was the only treatment available at that time. It is important to note that in this patient the diet was effective in the beginning and restored the young man to a state of maintaining healthy levels of blood sugar following the diet which, at the request of Dr Williams had been prescribed by Dr Francis Allen of New York.

However his condition gradually worsened and by 1920 he could only maintain a semblance of control by reducing his intake from 1900 calories a day, which he was having at the time of diagnosis, to less than 500 cal a day by the time he turned 20.

In 1922 around the time Banting was striving to try his extract, the 20-year-old Jim Havens was on less than 500 cal a day and weighed 74 pounds. His doctor felt defeated.

Needless to say, Williams was at the front of the queue to get some of Banting's extract. How he beat the competition provides an interesting and insightful story. It is probably one of many.

When Williams admitted his dilemma to his patient's father James S. Havens, a former congressman, the latter reached out to individuals all over the United States for help but to no avail. Then because he was the head of the legal department of the well-known Eastman Kodak Company he decided to see if any of his business contacts could help.

The manager of the Kodak store in Toronto did not have any direct information but said that his "golfing buddy" was a doctor. What's more the doctor worked at the Toronto General Hospital. The doctor's name was John J. A. Macleod.

Macleod mentioned that there was a group at the hospital working on an extract for diabetes and gave him Banting's name.

Banting, as had been his habit from the beginning, was generous with his sharing of the extract with doctors, sent some to Williams.

On May 17th, 1922 Williams injected some of Banting's extract into Havens. There was no clear improvement. When Banting heard this he immediately left Toronto with the supply of his extract and travelled directly to Rochester. Banting and Williams are said to have stayed awake all night, injecting the patient with insulin every two hours. This together with checking Jim's urine for sugar enabled the doctors to decide how much extract was needed to make the urine sugar-free. By the following morning Jim's urine was free of glucose and he was able to eat a full meal for lunch that day. Within one week he was feeling stronger and had started to do what he was keen on as a profession, drawing and painting.

On December 11, 1922 six months after Banting's mercy–dash from Toronto, Jim Havens wrote to the delighted Banting describing his treatment and his experience of eating eggs on toast for the first time in years saying that egg on toast was the "only food necessary in heaven."

Since insulin was still considered to be an "experimental drug" supplies had to cross the Canadian-American border secretly. Other challenges which accompanied the use of the early extracts included protein impurities which caused swelling and redness at the site of the injection.

Once again the superiority of the Lilly preparation was demonstrated when compared with the extract being made in Toronto.

By 1923 Lilly was producing insulin which had a higher potency with less irritation of the skin. However Lilly at that time was mostly producing pork insulin to which Havens was allergic.

In October 1923 Lilly started making beef insulin which proved to be much more suitable for him. Havens went on to become a skilful printer, painter and wood engraver. He married in 1927and had two children. Always interested in scientific advances in diabetes especially in insulin Havens had spent a considerable amount of time in Boston working with Elliott Joslin on experiments with insulin. Havens died of cancer in 1960.

Havens story illustrates several aspects of the development of insulin. It also provides another example of the difference between Banting and the other members of the team which discovered insulin. There is much criticism of Banting for various reasons but on one score he must be given his due. As mentioned before he was the only practising doctor in the entire group. His devotion to patients and his generosity with the insulin extract is demonstrated in this story by his journey to the patient's bedside. Banting staying awake all night together with the patient's doctor is the kind of story most doctors do not publicise but is commoner than is perhaps widely recognized.

THREE FAMOUS MEN SAVED BY INSULIN

The stories of these men, two American and the other English, who were saved by insulin and became famous for their contributions which diminished the suffering of other human beings, is a fitting conclusion to this part of the insulin story.

George Minot (1885–1950)

Minot, a medical graduate and son of Harvard professor, James Minot developed diabetes in 1921 when he was 36 years old. Standing 6'11/2 inches tall, Minot was an imposing athletic man held in high regard as a senior physician in Boston and soon to become Professor of Medicine at Harvard University.

Within weeks of developing diabetes Minot had lost weight. Being familiar with laboratory methods because of his research work as a haematologist he diagnosed his own condition and referred himself to Elliott Joslin. Diet being the only treatment available Joslin put him on 525 cal a day. Within weeks Minot's weight fell even further than the weight loss caused by diabetes which had brought him down from 147 to135 pounds. On the diet prescribed Minot's weight fell further to 120 pounds "and he looked it!"

Minot's wife was an exceptionally capable and attentive woman who grasped the basics of a diabetic diet quickly. They used to take a set of scales with them even when they went out to dinner in a restaurant and Marion knew the caloric value of every food item consumed by her husband. Little wonder then that his diabetic control was considered exemplary even by a physician as particular as Elliott Joslin.

As described earlier Joslin was very much in touch with advances in knowledge and treatment of diabetes even when such progress was in its nascent stages. He was, with Allen, among the first physicians in the United States to use insulin on his patients.

Minot started on insulin in January 1923. By 1924 he was on an injection before breakfast and at night. Marian reported that "this is the first winter since marriage that he has not lost 7 to 14 days from his illness."

Minot went on to a distinguished career in medicine specialising in haematology. In 1934 he was awarded the Nobel Prize in Physiology or Medicine together with William Murphy and George Whipple for discovering the treatment for Pernicious Anaemia.

Minot lived for nearly 30 years, taking insulin every day.

The famous haematologist William Castle commented that Banting's and Best's discovery of insulin in 1921 not only transformed diabetes treatment but also, by keeping Minot alive, contributed towards the discovery of a cure for Pernicious Anaemia.

When I met Charles Best many years later in 1969, one of the things he told me about his association with Dr Elliott Joslin was the latter's advice to him to "develop a habit of keeping in touch with your patients long–term because that's how you will learn how diabetes behaves."

During my preparation for this book I found a reference to George Minot in the Best family papers as recorded by Henry Best in his book *Margaret and Charlie*.

In the summer of 1927, during a driving holiday which took them to Boston, Charles Best and his wife had lunch with Dr and Mrs George Minot. Their diary recorded the following,

"Minot, a severe diabetic, collaborated with George H.Whipple and William P. Murphy in the discovery of the liver treatment for Pernicious Anaemia. Proud of Minot's achievement, Best nominated him and Whipple for the Nobel Prize, which they shared with Murphy in 1934."

Robert Daniel Lawrence (1892–1968)

"I've got insulin – it works – come back quick"
                                        Cable sent to Lawrence in May 1923

A brilliant student and excellent sportsman Robert "Robin" Lawrence developed severe diabetes in 1920. At that time developing diabetes was tantamount to receiving a death sentence. Thinking he only had a short time to live, Lawrence did not wish to die at home which would have been distressing to his family. He therefore moved to Florence in Tuscany and set up a practice there. In the European winter of 1922–23 his diabetes became much worse after an attack of a chest infection. He was sure that the end was near.

When news of the discovery of insulin by Banting and colleagues in Toronto hit the headlines in Europe and England Lawrence's ex-chief at the hospital in London (Kings College) where he had worked before moving to Italy, cabled him saying "I've got insulin...... come back quick."

Lawrence left immediately and drove across the continent to reach Kings College hospital on 28th of May 1923. He was very weak and and his condition was made worse by painful legs because of neuritis which is often seen in patients with untreated diabetes.

His first insulin injection was on 31 May 1923. He spent two months in hospital recovering and spent all that time learning about insulin. He devoted the rest of his life to the care of diabetic patients. His instruction manual for diabetic patients which was inspired by the pioneer of education for diabetic patients, Elliott Joslin of Boston, went to seventeen editions. Together with the famous English novelist H.G.Wells, also a diabetic, who was his patient, Lawrence started the British Diabetic Association which continues to serve the diabetic community to this day.

Lawrence, saved by insulin, lived for over 40 years and died in 1968 at the age of 76.

Randall G Sprague

Born in 1906, Sprague was 16 years old at the time of the discovery of insulin. He had developed diabetes a few months before the discovery and had rapidly lost weight. He was weak and wasted with a body weight of 78 pounds when his parents brought him to the well-known physician Rollin Woodyatt. After inconsistent results with the extracts developed in Woodyatt's laboratory, Sprague was eventually satisfactorily stabilised on the preparation obtained from the Lilly laboratories.

He worked at the renowned Mayo Clinic in Rochester and became a prominent physician and a leader in the American medical fraternity. He had specialised in treating diabetes and was a great advocate for education in the treatment of diabetic patients as pioneered by Elliott Joslin of Boston since the early 1900s.

Sprague was in excellent condition when contacted by Michael Bliss for the book published in 1982. He told Bliss that he had lived a healthy life for 60 years and estimated that he had injected himself 45,000 times with insulin.

Teddy Ryder the Story of One of "The Four Living Skeletons"

In July 1922 supplies of insulin extract were proving a challenge because of the unreliability of their production. During this time Banting, who was alone because Best had gone on holidays, received one batch of insulin from the Connaught Laboratories and decided to treat four particularly emaciated patients, three children and one adult. The story of one of these patients was recorded as a footnote at the end of Bliss's book which was published in 1982, sixty years after the incident involving the "four living skeletons".

One of the three children treated by Banting was Teddy Ryder who was five years old at that time. His weight was 26 pounds (11.8 kg). He had received his first insulin injection from Banting on July 10, 1922. In 1983 the patient who had taken insulin injections for 61 years, was free of complications and living in retirement in Connecticut. His mother recalled that on her way to Toronto in 1922 she had overheard a passerby commenting on her little boy, "She will never bring that child back alive."

The mother, still alive at 92, had never forgotten that trip in the summer of 1922 or "the wonderful Doctor Banting."

INSULIN FOR THE WORLD

The difficulties encountered with the use of the extract prepared by Banting and Best on Leonard Thompson on 11 January, 1922 had been bitterly disappointing especially for Banting. So it was a huge relief when better results were obtained when the extract prepared by Collip was given to the same patient.

Collip's lapse which was entirely unexpected and unforeseen and remains a mystery to this day, was followed by a six-week period in mid–May to June 1922 (after Collip had left Toronto) when Best and his colleagues including John Hepburn developed an effective method for large-scale production of insulin. They were now in a position to provide "purified"insulin to meet the clinical and experimental needs in Toronto for the next three months. Clearly the manufacturing of insulin for the needs of diabetics beyond Toronto or even Canada was going to require considerable expansion of the facilities for its manufacture.

The large-scale insulin production by Best and his team was carried out in the Connaught Antitoxin Laboratories.

This institution played a central role in the discovery of insulin by Banting and Best as did it's director John Fitzgerald. The history of both the Connaught Laboratories and Fitzgerald are of interest and relevance to the insulin story.

The Connaught Antitoxin Laboratories.

These laboratories were situated on a farm on the outskirts of Toronto. The land had been donated by Colonel Albert Gooderham, a scion of one of the wealthiest families in Toronto and the owner of a whiskey distillery firm he had inherited from his father in 1905. The Gooderham name was prominent in Toronto's commercial history from as far back as the early 1800s. A newspaper article singing the praises of the Gooderham dynasty said, "every time you turn you would have another story about the Gooderham impact on the city. The Toronto Symphony Orchestra, Bank of Toronto, King Edward hotel, Connaught Antitoxin Laboratories, hospitals and life insurance companies, all had Gooderham connections."

The founder of the Antitoxin Laboratories was John "Jerry" Fitzgerald. In all the published accounts of the insulin story Fitzgerald is very much in the background. However he played a critical role not only in the commercial development of insulin but also in the lives of the insulin team especially Banting and Best. A brief account of his background is useful when one looks at his contributions to the insulin story.

John Gerald "Jerry" Fitzgerald (1882–1940) was the son of William Fitzgerald, a pharmacist. His paternal ancestors were Irish who had emigrated from County Monaghan in the Republic of Ireland to Upper Canada in 1824.

Jerry was born in Drayton. The family moved to Harristown in 1891. During his high school years Jerry worked as an apprentice in his father's apothecary store. He also helped care for his invalid mother.

Fitzgerald entered the University of Toronto faculty of medicine in 1899. At 16 he was the youngest in his class. He graduated in 1903 aged 21. A family history of mental instability led Fitzgerald to study the biological roots of insanity first in Buffalo New York, and later, Johns Hopkins where he was inspired by the leading figure in American public health, William Henry Welch.

In 1907 he was a Clinical Director of the Toronto Asylum for the Insane. In 1909 after a year at Harvard, and a change of direction, he switched to study bacteriology.

In 1907 he married a wealthy heiress Edna Leonard. During the honeymoon while travelling in Europe, Fitzgerald worked with Emile Roux at the Pasteur Institute. Roux (1853 –1933) was one of the closest collaborators of Louis Pasteur (1822–1895). Fitzgerald was probably taken by but certainly agreed with one of Pasteur's well known aphorisms,

"Let me tell you the secret that has led me to my goal. My strengths lies solely in my tenacity."

Also, "science knows no country, because knowledge belongs to humanity and is the torch with illuminates the world."

Between 1910 and 1913 Fitzgerald sacrificed all vacations and engaged in an intensive study of bacteriology and pathology. He was befriended by leading international scientists including Elie Metchnikoff, the father of immunology. Fitzgerald also established a lifelong friendship with Emile Roux.

During this period Fitzgerald learned how to make the vaccines pioneered by Pasteur including rabies vaccine, diphtheria antitoxin and smallpox vaccine.

Upon his return to Toronto in 1913 he was appointed Associate Professor in the newly formed Department of Hygiene.

Fitzgerald's vision was to reform public health in Canada. Thousands were dying from infectious disease. Diphtheria alone was a leading killer of children under 14. Antitoxins and vaccines were all imported from the United States at prohibitively high prices.

In 1913 soon after Fitzgerald had arrived in Toronto, he approached the Toronto University Board of Governors with a proposal to set up a laboratory in the Department of Hygiene to manufacture high-quality preventive medicines at costs low enough to make them universally available –"within reach of everyone."

Then, without waiting for the university's approval, the 30-year-old dynamic and driven young reformer went out on his own. Borrowing from his wife's inheritance, Fitzgerald aquired five horses which were destined for the knackery and boarded them in a small stable he built on Barton Avenue, one of the backstreets near the university. The horses were injected with toxins of diphtheria and in this way he produced Canada's first antitoxin for the condition. The project also demonstrated the feasibility of his proposal.

The governors of the university's board required no further proof of the capability and determination of the young scientist, nor his noble and altruistic principles.

The Antitoxin Laboratories were launched on 1 May, 1914 in the basement of the Toronto University medical school. However it was self– supporting and received no funds from the University. Public subscriptions supported the institution largely because of the reputation of the young scientist chosen to be in charge. Interestingly one of the public donors was Edmund Boyd Osler, brother of the famous Canadian physician William Osler. Edmund Osler's contribution helped to establish a space dedicated to a general laboratory, a sterilising facility and a small bacteriological laboratory. The outbreak of the 1914–1918 World War a few months later required the services of the newly established laboratory to immunise the troops against tetanus.

Fitzgerald's brilliance coupled with persistence and courage had not gone unnoticed. A philanthropist and a third – generation whiskey distiller by the name of Albert Edward Gooderham who had noticed the 30-year-old professor's drive, donated 58 acres of land north-west of Toronto together with buildings and funds to expand the Antitoxin laboratory which at Gooderham's request were called the "Connaught Antitoxin Laboratories" after a recent Governor General of Canada, the Duke of Connaught who also happened to be the youngest son of the English monarch Queen Victoria. Some of the work on the search for insulin was carried out on these premises.

Returning to the festering disquiet and discord between Banting and Macleod one can understand that given his background, Fitzgerald's sympathies may have been with Banting. Like Fitzgerald, Banting had always put the interests of the patient first.

Fitzgerald would have wondered about Macleod's role in the insulin project not only because of his participation as a fellow-scientist but also as the Head of the Department of Physiology and more importantly, the Dean of the Faculty of Medicine. Macleod and Fitzgerald were around the same age. Both had laboratory and clinical experience and held positions of administration and authority at the University. Fitzgerald certainly would have understood Banting's frustrations and perhaps, without sharing this with Banting, wondered about Macleod's approach to his various roles and responsibilities in relation to the insulin experiments. Was Macleod the leader, the fellow-researcher, or the guide? Or was he, as believed by Banting, a rival scheming to take credit for work done by another.

Fitzgerald realised that the continuing friction between Banting and Macleod might be resolved by a senior man respected by the community, namely Gooderham. Given Fitzgerald's well known belief in the practice of providing medical relief at no cost, he wanted the wise counsel of a man better versed in matters of money and profit. Doubtless he would have been disappointed in the most senior member of the insulin research group failing to provide leadership to the younger men who may have been looking at financial gain from what was clearly a life-saving treatment for thousands around the world.

Fitzgerald had provided funds allocated to the Connaught Antitoxin laboratories for equipment to be used by the insulin team when they began working towards large-scale production of insulin.

To an observer it may appear that Fitzgerald, rather than Macleod, was providing the leadership needed at this stage for the younger men including Banting to work as a team to produce insulin.

Banting was drawn to Fitzgerald by the latter's many qualities especially his altruism and integrity. The young researcher had recognised in Fitzgerald virtues which he felt were absent in Macleod. Their friendship continued to the end of Fitzgerald's life.

When Fitzgerald died in tragic circumstances – he took his own life at the age of 58 – Banting asked Best to accompany him as one of the pallbearers of the brilliant and altruistic scientist.

Gooderham the failed Peacemaker

A major hurdle in the developmental phase of insulin came to a head towards the end of the summer of 1922. Best had started his medical studies in September. At the same time he was continuing with his work at the Connaught laboratories as the Head of the insulin production team which required frequent out-of-town visits mostly to the production facilities of Eli Lilly Company in Indianapolis.

The strained relationship between Macleod and Banting worsened when Macleod refused to correct published accounts in newspapers attributing major credit to him as the most senior man in the group and the Head of the department where the work had taken place. Macleod, instead of correcting such statements remained silent which appeared, at least to Banting, to let the misconception persist. This led to Banting making a statement which was published in the *Toronto Star* on September 9, 1922.

"It would appear from articles that have appeared in some papers that Mr Best was not associated with me in my research work until after some progress had been made. I would like to correct that impression. Mr Best was with me from the first. The idea came to me in November 1920, while I was on the staff of the Western University, London, Ontario. In May 1921, Mr Best and I made the first experiment and we have been working together ever since.

While the idea, it is true, is mine, Mr Best must have equal credit for the success we have attained. I never would have been able to do anything had it not been for him. We have worked together side by side, sharing ideas and developing them together, and but for his unflagging devotion and his enthusiasm and his patient and meticulous work we would never have made the progress we have.

From the very beginning it has been a case of Banting and Best and if our hopes are realised I desire to see Mr Best given all the honour that will be his due."

In an attempt to resolve the impasse Fitzgerald, as the Head of Connaught Laboratories, turned to his friend Colonel Albert Gooderham.

The choice of Gooderham as mediator by Fitzgerald was an example of his "people skills" on the one hand and the ability to manage bureaucracy on the other. Gooderham was the Chairman of the Insulin Committee of the University of Toronto Board of Governors.

He asked Banting, Best and Macleod to provide an individual statement of their understanding of their contributions to the discovery of insulin from the very beginning to the current stage of production. Gooderham told them that he hoped to reach a consensus based on their statements after examining the differences in the statement of the three participants.

Macleod submitted a six–page report.

Banting summarised his dissatisfaction in six points which included "a lack of trust and co-operation on the part of Professor Macleod." He pointed to Macleod repeatedly trying to appropriate credit which rightly belonged to Banting and to some extent, also to Best.

Best's report was the shortest stating that "conversations with Dr. Banting and Dr. Macleod" made further comment unnecessary.

Commenting on Best's brief report Henry Best in his book attributed it to the long hours Best was spending in the laboratory.

In later years Dr Barbara Hazlett, in a textbook on diabetes published in 2000, *Clinical Diabetes Mellitus: A Problem-Oriented Approach* by John K. Davidson wrote,

"Best wrote a fair account, giving credit to Macleod for suggesting alcohol extraction and immediate chilling, and to Collip for determining the highest concentration of alcohol in which the active principle was soluble. She added, "the relationships between the four men are the most interesting – jealousy, greed, paranoia, and innocence, intermingled with hard work in dreadful conditions and brilliance."

Possibly the technical aspects of the situation described in the statement were too much for the whiskey magnate but whatever the reason, Gooderham failed to achieve any kind of reconciliation. The animosity between Banting and Macleod was never resolved.

By early July 1922 the commercial production of insulin was being carried out in Toronto at the antitoxin laboratories with Charles Best having been made its director on January 1, 1922 even though he was still in the middle of his studies. He did not submit his MA thesis till May 1 of that year.

Banting had been appointed to head the Diabetic Clinic attached to Christie Street Military Hospital. This position had been created specially for Banting because of difficulties in getting an appointment to Toronto General Hospital. Later in the year the stubborn Duncan Graham was prevailed upon to grant Banting a position to treat patients there as documented in a letter to the President of the University of Toronto. The circumstances of this incident are described below. The establishment of the diabetic clinic attached to the Christie Street hospital provided Banting with a facility for treating diabetics. The letter of that appointment was dated April 8, 1922. He had started using insulin produced in the Connaught laboratories and had commented that he was "treating skeletons."

As for Banting's access to Toronto General, once again it was in all likelihood Macleod who had persuaded Graham to relent as far as Banting was concerned because it was becoming increasingly awkward for the Head of the Department of Physiology which had put itself at the forefront of the production team after the success of the injections of the extract prepared by Collip to explain Banting's absence from the team using insulin. The situation for Graham was even more awkward because having earlier blocked Banting's attempts to work at the hospital he could hardly allow any other member of the team given that Banting was the only medically qualified individual in the research group.

The two Scotsmen Macleod and Graham realised too late that each had badly misjudged the situation and had failed to see the bigger picture.

They were taken aback by the blunt and awkward questions levelled at Graham by none other than the Chairman of the hospital's Board of Trustees, C. W. Blackwell. Blackwell, who had been on a trip to visit American hospitals, was repeatedly asked about the results of using insulin at the hospital attached to the university where the magic potion had been discovered. One phone call to Graham revealed the embarrassing fact that insulin was not in use in the hospital and also that Banting was not on the staff. Blackwell had found that most people regarded Banting as the principal discoverer of insulin.

He was livid. It didn't take him long to discover the obstructive tactics used by Graham to block Banting's repeated attempts at securing a clinical appointment to conduct the trials of the extract on Leonard Thompson in January of that year.

Blackwell ignored Graham and went straight to the President of the University, Sir Robert Falconer.

The Scotsman's intransigence was coming back to bite him. He was asked why Banting, the only doctor in the team which discovered insulin, was not allowed to treat patients in the hospital attached to the University where his research had taken place.

Yes, Campbell was the Head Physician at Toronto General but as D.E. Robertson, another physician, had said to Duncan Graham, "Campbell knows all about diabetes but cannot treat it and Banting knows nothing about diabetes but *can* treat it."

Falconer's main concern was the reputation of the university. He was conscious of the possibility that with all the attempts mainly by Graham at the hospital and Macleod at university to keep Banting out could result in American physicians, who were already more experienced in treating diabetics then their Canadian cousins, making it possible for American diabetics to get insulin in preference to Canadians. That would reflect badly on the whole country. Falconer realised the importance of resolving this potentially embarrassing situation as soon as possible and bluntly told Graham to rectify it.

An ad hoc university committee chaired by Falconer himself met in mid June with the aim of resolving the infighting and to ensure that Banting would have not only an appointment at the hospital but also at the University. In one fell swoop the President of the University had made the best-laid plans of both Scotsmen irrelevant.

The letter from the chastened Chairman of the Department of Medicine submitted to Sir Robert Falconer was dated July 20, 1922. This was after insulin from Toronto had been used on patients in other cities including in the United States where on May 22nd, 1922 a young man called Jim Havens under the care of the well-known endocrinologist of Rochester Dr J.R. Williams had become the first American to receive insulin.

The letter read as follows:

"Dear Sir Robert,

I'm enclosing a memorandum with reference to the recommended hospital arrangements and staff appointments for the diabetic clinic in order that you may be kept posted of the progress we are making.

We discussed the enclosed memorandum with Mr Blackwell* this morning. They have accepted the recommendations made and we hope to begin the treatment of cases, both private and public, on or about August 15.

I should like to call your attention to the arrangements made with reference to Doctors Campbell and Fletcher. As the organisation of the Diabetic Clinic is a temporary one it was considered best that both doctors Campbell and Fletcher should continue with their present private practice. It will be necessary for Dr. Campbell to give up his present whole time appointment in the Department of Medicine for the coming year. On your return in September I should recommend that Dr. Campbell be appointed a Senior Demonstrator on a part time basis and that Dr. Banting be appointed a Senior

Demonstrator in Medicine on a part-time basis, and Junior
Assistant Attending Physician to the Toronto General Hospital.
I trust these recommendations will meet with your approval.
With kindest regards, I am,
Yours sincerely
(signed) Duncan Graham"
Professor of Medicine.

The embarrassment caused by Duncan Graham's refusal to afford
Banting clinical privileges at the hospital remains an unfortunate
chapter in the history of the discovery of insulin.

As if this weren't enough further incidents of pettiness were
to emerge during this early period after the discovery had become
public. Once again, the more mature and sensible individuals
like Fitzgerald had to intervene to salvage the reputation of the
University and, given the international publicity of the discovery,
the reputation of not only Toronto but Canada.

The Scientific Community's Response to the Discovery
Oscar Minkowski's Reaction

It is appropriate to begin this part of the story with the reaction
of the man who occupied, and continues to occupy a pride of
place in discoveries relating to diabetes. Oscar Minkowski had
recognised and had proved that the pancreas was the seat of
diabetes even though he had been unable to produce an effective
extract of insulin. His reaction was described in an essay written
by Martin Goldner who went on to become a prominent
diabetologist in America after completing his training. Goldner
was in Breslow in the spring of 1923 when as a medical student he
attended a regular morning lecture by Professor Minkowski. The
popular professor showed the students the first vial of insulin sent
to Germany by Banting and Best. Minkowski said to his students,
"it was once my hope that I would be the father of insulin. Now
I'm happy to accept the designation as it's grandfather, which the
Toronto scientists have conferred on me so kindly."

Goldner went on to say that many of the students that morning felt that they had witnessed a historical moment and had seen the old professor's gracious acknowledgement that his life's aim had been fulfilled by the ingenious research of younger men, but had also witnessed the dawn of a new era in the treatment of diabetes..."

The scientist in Minkowski however, could not suppress his observation on a critical and technical aspect of the experiments which had facilitated the Torontonians' success. Minkowski pointed out that improvements in the method of measuring glucose levels in the blood had played an important part in the discovery. The new method developed by chemists including S.R. Benedict and Folin in the early 1900s had made it possible for blood glucose levels to be measured more quickly. Furthermore the new method had the added advantage of needing much smaller samples of blood.

The Skepticism of Two Respected Doctors

Given the history of the leadership provided by prominent German scientists and teachers, under normal circumstances there would have been great interest amongst them in the discovery of insulin and following that, its manufacture. However in the aftermath of the 1914–1918 war, Germany had other priorities dominated by rebuilding virtually every sector of its industries.

The highly influential diabetes specialist Carl von Noorden is said to have tried insulin on his patients towards the end of 1922 but had discarded the practice of using it because of its short-lived effect on the reduction of blood glucose levels and it's failure to clear the urine of glucose. Von Noorden had a very large number of patients with diabetes and was a respected clinician and teacher on the condition.

Bernhardt Naunyn (1839-1925), was the author of the widely used German diabetes text "Der Diabetes Melitus" (*sic*) published in 1898. He was also a teacher and a mentor of many American physicians including Elliott Joslin and Graham Lusk.

Naunyn had reservations. In a letter to Minkowski, Naunyn then in his 80s, said that he was sceptical. He considered the reports on insulin an example of "American exaggeration".

The British Response

To say that Toronto, or for that matter even Canada, did not occupy a position of prominence in the international scientific community when compared with the traditional centres of scientific research or teaching would be an understatement. Neither the city nor the country would have been mentioned in the same breath as Germany, France or England. Closer to home, the American academic institutions like Harvard, Yale and Johns Hopkins were in a different league altogether.

It was therefore not surprising that within months of hearing about the discovery of insulin in the summer of 1922, Britain sent two of its leading scientists, Henry Dale and Harold Dudley from the National Institute for Medical Research "to report on the progress of this remarkable discovery and on the initial results of its practical application......"

The duo arrived in Toronto in the autumn of 1922. The assessment according to Charles Best was an accurate reflection of the stage of progress in the discovery and development of insulin up to that point. This quote is from the Joslin archives of records kept by Charles Best.

"We arrived in Toronto towards the end of September and the evidence put before us carried immediate conviction that a genuine discovery of great potential importance had been made...

Professor James J.R. Macleod had organised a team of workers to reinforce the activities of the original discoverers in work directed to the improvement of methods for estimating the amount of insulin present in extracts, and to the production of purer preparations in a higher yield. The practical production was, indeed still (is), in its infancy."

Apart from Macleod, Dale did not name any other members of the team. This is at odds with the recollections of Charles Best in his later years when he claimed that Dale had said that it was Best who had the clearest understanding of the whole situation relating to the discovery of insulin.

Dale's assessment clarifies that the Torontonians were at this stage well past the point of the discovery of insulin and had moved on to the next phase namely the development of insulin.

It is important to appreciate the foresight of Fred Banting in recognising the importance of education in the use of insulin not only for the patient but also by other members of the treatment team such as the parents of children with diabetes, as well as the associated medical team including nurses, dieticians and last, but not least, the treating physicians.

Interestingly, Charles Best's father, Dr. Herbert Best, who was a general practitioner in Maine, made arrangements to come to Toronto to learn about diabetes and how to treat it with insulin. Charles Best, who was not even in medical school at that time, arranged for one of the physicians at the Toronto General Hospital, Dr. Roscoe to take his father under his wing. Roscoe, according to Charles Best, treated the senior man with great respect.

Reality Check! Charles Best's and Toronto's Limitations in Insulin Production

The insulin production team was led by Charles Best. This particular appointment was to have an unforeseen influence on the young graduate in the immediate future and which persisted throughout his life.

To Banting and Best were added Bertram Collip (for the first few weeks), John Hepburn, J.K. Latchford, N.A. McCormick, and Clark Noble.

The insulin production team, for the first time, included only one (Best) of the two original researchers because Banting, as noted previously, prioritised using insulin to treat patients in Toronto (including those who came to Toronto), and also to developing a teaching program designed to instruct patients and physicians in the clinical application of insulin. By training, and at heart, Banting was always a clinician and not a researcher.

Collip had only stayed a few weeks while Macleod continued in a largely administrative role and dealt with various interested parties including pharmaceutical companies like Lilly and individuals like Allen and Joslin.

Technical assistance with the production of a suitable extract was almost entirely obtained from the research personnel of the Lilly laboratories.

The appointment of Charles Best as the head of the production team working in the Connaught laboratories is puzzling. The thinking behind Best's appointment has never been explained or for that matter explored, let alone questioned. He was still a university student and his lack of experience is clear from all the accounts of the discovery of insulin described in various documents and books including this one.

In short, Best, had no experience except that which he had gained in the laboratory as an undergraduate. That work was general and not related to the work on insulin which he had undertaken as a laboratory assistant to Banting over the summer months of 1921.

The other very important aspect of producing insulin was the need to meet the challenges of its distribution to the wider community beyond Toronto and indeed throughout the world. Best was entirely lacking in training let alone experience in the competitive cut-throat world of the commercial aspects such as sales and distribution of any pharmaceutical product let alone an entirely new one which was so urgently needed and sought throughout the world.

It soon became clear that the local production in Toronto was going to be insufficient even for local needs.

Given the earlier hurdles Banting had to overcome it was ironic that once insulin was being produced at Connaught, more than 2/3 of it went to Banting because of his dual appointments to Toronto General Hospital as well as the Christie Street Clinic for treatment of veterans. Given his commitment and loyalty to his friends it was not surprising that Joe Gilchrist was appointed as a physician at the Christie Street facility.

Banting was devoting the rest of his time to organising programs for teaching patients as well as physicians the practical aspects of the use of insulin. In this regard he was frequently in touch with one of the leading clinicians in diabetes in that part of the world, namely Elliott Joslin of Boston.

When Banting Wept

Banting's new commitments meant that Charles Best no longer had the constant companionship of Fred Banting, who had been so loyal in the immediate aftermath of the discovery of insulin by including Best in all the acknowledgement and praise heaped upon him (Banting) by the press, politicians, supporters and friends.

Banting had used his influence and new found fame to raise funds for additional equipment for the Connaught Laboratories. In the early stages of manufacture he had gone to Indianapolis himself on a few occasions.

An oft-repeated story tells of Banting's sensitivity on the matter of "owning"the results of the research on insulin which had made him suspicious of the motives of the Lilly company shortly after the two parties, largely through the persistence and foresight of Lilly's J.H.A. Clowse, had joined forces to produce insulin on a larger scale. Thinking Lilly might be keeping some secret to themselves Banting went to meet the Lilly executives only to find that the owner Josiah K. Lilly himself was there to meet him. Disarmed by the warmth of his welcome in Indianapolis to say nothing of the Southern hospitality – remember that the founder of Lilly, Colonel Eli Lilly, had started his working life as a plantation manager in the south–Banting was overcome when the company gave him all the information he wanted together with a much larger supply of insulin than he had dreamed of.

The head of the company Josiah K. Lilly wrote to his son Eli about the meeting with Banting.

"When they left Toronto, there was not a single unit left in the city. Banting ..... has a large number of patients, and he certainly was in trouble. We had 150 units ready for him, and when I told him he could take it back with him, he fell on my shoulder and wept, and when I told him that the next evening we would send him 150 units, he was transported into the realms of bliss. Banting is really a fine chap and we must back him to the limit."

Macleod Outclassed

If the assistance of Lilly Company was invaluable for Charles Best it was also a lifeline for Macleod. Inexperienced in commercial matters he was haunted by the fear of other laboratories succeeding in isolating insulin from the pancreas as had been described by the Toronto team in medical journals and, thanks to the lay press, in magazine articles. Worse still if such a company were to take out a patent on the discovery there was a potential for exploitation of patients unable to afford the price of insulin.

Within weeks of starting production it became clear that the Connaught laboratories did not have the capacity for producing more than a small amount of insulin. Therefore a letter from Clowse of Lilly in March 1922 may well have made Macleod heave a sigh of relief. The canny Englishman who assured Macleod of his firm's continued interest in developing the extract discovered by Macleod's team, had sensed the inexperienced academic's apprehensions. Clowse fuelled the physiologist's fear by referring to the possibility of

".....attempts on the part of unprincipled individuals to victimise the public..."

He urged Macleod to reconsider the decision not to work with a major manufacturing firm before delivering what would have made it clear to the academic that he and his team were novices in the uncharted waters of commercial competition. In other words the huge gap in experience and resources between the pharmaceutical giant Lilly and the fledgeling "manufacturers" at Connaught was obvious.

Clowes went further saying, "I have this far refrained from starting working on laboratories as I was anxious to avoid in any way intruding on the field of yourself and your associates until you had published your results. I feel, however, that the matter is now one of such immediate importance that we should take up the experimental end of the question without delay, preferably cooperating with you and your associates...."

In other words, Clowse made it clear to Macleod that if he didn't agree, Lilly could proceed without Toronto's cooperation.

A Historic Commercial Arrangement May 22nd 1922

Clowse was invited to come to Toronto on May 22nd, 1922.

An interesting associated account highlights the difference between the academic and financially inexperienced – even naive – members of the medical fraternity, versus the hard-nosed commercial practitioners.

At the same time as they had invited the Lilly research director, the Torontonians had also invited the well-known and respected American physician Rollin Woodyatt. This was intended to signal to the pharmaceutical firm that they were in competition with another interested party.

Woodyatt of Chicago had offered the services of his expert staff whose expertise and competence was respected throughout the United States, together with the assurance of financial backing and, as a sweetener, the pancreas resources of the Chicago stockyards. There was just one problem. Woodyatt's work commitments to his academic, research and treatment of patients in the office and hospital did not allow him to come to Toronto on the appointed date of May 22nd, 1922.

By contrast, Clowse who had been ensconced in the luxury suites of the King Edward Hotel (owned by, the Gooderham family) did not only arrive at the appointed time but came accompanied by a team from his firm to meet with Fitzgerald, Macleod and Best. The three academics were taken aback to see Clowse approaching with three other men. They were a senior chemist of the firm, a patent attorney, and the Vice President of Eli Lilly namely Mr Eli Lilly, the son of Josiah Lilly, the President and owner of the firm. To say that there was an imbalance in knowledge and experience of commercial matters between the two teams would be an understatement. However, the negotiations were completed courteously and seamlessly largely because of the sophisticated and practised approach of the commercially savvy team of the pharmaceutical firm.

In a formal letter to Sir Robert Falconer, Fitzgerald acknowledged the limitations of the research team.

"Experience in the production of insulin on a moderately large scale in the Connaught Laboratories has shown that this is fraught with many difficulties ...and we do not believe that production in amounts that are adequate to supply the demands for it can be accomplished without further experimentation on a much larger scale. To make this further step possible it will be necessary for us to collaborate with some well-equipped and properly staffed commercial house which is engaged in this work.

We have chosen to collaborate with Eli Lilly and Company."

Fitzgerald also stated that the group would publish in full the details of the method used in Toronto at the Connaught laboratories so that other concerns including smaller establishments such as hospitals and non-commercial companies would be free to develop their own supplies.

The formalisation of the agreement brought to a satisfactory conclusion the overtures first made by Clowse to Macleod after the very first "public" presentation by Banting and Best at the Department of Physiology Journal Club on 14 November, 1921.

The Lilly Company A Brief History

The Lilly Company is one of, if not the oldest, companies which have supplied insulin worldwide from 1922 to the present day. A brief history of the company highlights the many differences between it and Connaught Laboratories especially in the scale of operations for the manufacture of products.

At the time of the joining of forces, the Lilly Company had been in operation for nearly 50 years having started in May 1876. By the late 1880s it had more than 100 employees and was generating $200,000 in annual sales. At the time of joining with Connaught Laboratories in the insulin venture, the Lilly Company was being run by the son of the founder. Josiah Lilly added several technological advances to the manufacturing process and significantly, a research and manufacturing plant, the Lilly Biological Laboratories. This was built in 1913.

In 1919 Josiah Lilly hired a biochemist and medical graduate called George Henry Clowse (1877–1958) as Director of Research. In addition to his new employee's scientific knowledge and experience Lilly had detected an additional asset in the Englishman, a shrewd business brain.

Thus in terms of history, personnel and financial clout the company which had joined forces with the fledgeling group charged with producing insulin in Toronto was in a different class in every way.

George Walden, a Chemist's Chemist

Following the formalisation of the agreement between Lilly and the Toronto team, Clowse encouraged both Banting and Best to visit the facilities in Indianapolis. This resulted in several improvements in the equipment being used at the Connaught Laboratories. The changes were largely based on the improvements already in place in the Lilly laboratories through the expertise of George Walden, the chief chemist whom Clowse had given the insulin project. As the head of that division the Englishman had impressed on Walden the importance of insulin which he could see had market potential like no other pharmaceutical product at that time.

Walden, unlike the other chemists engaged in refining the insulin extract, made an intensive study of the work on insulin up to that point. After familiarising himself with published material in scientific journals plus information gained, largely through Clowes's practice of keeping his ear to the ground for any information on promising pharmaceuticals, Walden spent a great deal of time examining every step of the production and purification of insulin used in Toronto.

The breakthrough came when Walden discovered the critical step dealing with the acidity of different batches of extract. He found that the acidity varied from batch to batch. This explained the different and unpredictable effects of injecting the extract into diabetic animals in the laboratory as well as in human patients. Walden was able to correct this and produce a stable and reliable product suitable for treatment of diabetes. Walden's methodical and patient approach allowed the Lilly Company to be ahead of its competitors especially in Britain.

Two Englishman at Loggerheads

The involvement of the Connaught Laboratories with the Lilly Company was timely. It had become increasingly clear to the comparatively small group of workers at Connaught including Charles Best that the production of the extract in quantities sufficient for the needs even locally in Toronto to supply the hospital and Fred Banting's clinic was proving a challenge as indicated in the comment by Josiah Lilly above.

Charles Best, at the time of leaving for his summer holidays in July 1922, called the situation of extract production at Connaught "a nightmare." There were numerous problems with local complications of infection and allergic reactions at the site of injections and, more worryingly, the unpredictability of the effectiveness of the extract from one batch to the next. Whatever they tried simply did not work.

One might observe that it would have been thought unusual for the head of a concern like the Connaught Laboratories to go on holidays leaving behind unresolved problems at the laboratory. Was this indicative of a lack of experience on the part of Best or was it due to being over-committed with his plans to start medical studies while continuing in the role of the leader of the team charged with the task of large-scale Insulin production at Connaught.

Clowse kept his promise and shared Walden's findings with the inexperienced chemists in the team at Toronto.

He did not however share any "trade secrets" with the chemists in England where the work was largely directed by Henry Dale. In some quarters it was felt that there was little love lost between the two Englishmen.

Dale who had worked for a time at the British drug company Burroughs Wellcome was suspicious of the motives of the Lilly operative. The personal rivalry between the two Englishmen was a source of amusement for the American employers of Clowse.

Dale felt that the Toronto team had played into the hands of the commercially driven pharmaceutical company. In a letter to Fletcher, the physician at Toronto General Hospital, Dale referred to the Toronto team as "those blundering amateurs." In spite of the many obstacles and behind-the-scenes manoeuvring the end result of the tug-of-war between Lilly and the different interested parties, starting with Connaught Laboratories and then the English was a victory for the pharmaceutical company. The strategy used by Clowse was one of cooperation, even compromise as long as Lilly was able to get the other parties to agree to the Indianapolis company manufacturing insulin on a large scale. This was because it had become clear to Clowse that compared to Lilly his competitors in Toronto and Britain were minnows.

The end result of the various commercial negotiations saw Lilly become the leading supplier of insulin not only in the United States but in most countries of the world. In its first year of marketing it sold more than $1 million worth of insulin and its financial future looked golden. We will meet this company in "the same but different" guise later in this story.

Charles Best and the Fringe Benefits of His New Position

In the summer of 1922 Best made nearly a dozen trips to Indianapolis. There are few details of knowledge gained through the study of the methods in use in the laboratory under the supervision of Walden. What Best described in detail especially in his letters to Margaret Mahon were the opulent hotel rooms reserved for him and paid for by Lilly. On one occasion he mentioned the hotel Lincoln with "450 rooms and 450 baths!" This is before he had seen the palatial home of the owner Josiah Lilly. It is also well known that Clowse himself was an ardent collector of art. Whether Best was invited to the Clowes home is not documented but clearly the young man was wined and dined to such an extent that he needed little encouragement to visit the Lilly facilities.

At the end of 1922 Charles Best went home to Maine for Christmas. He spent one day in Montréal where he visited the Montréal General and Royal Victoria hospitals. He said, "insulin is a magic word. The man in charge of the diabetics, Dr. Rabinowich (he needs no other description) nearly turned himself inside out to entertain us. We toured the hospital, lunched there and eventually rode in a prepaid cab to the Royal Vic. Mason is the man in charge there. He had received several impotent lots of "Isletin" and was a bit sceptical at first, but thawed and gave us a very busy and interesting afternoon."

These accounts cast a light on some of the experiences Charles Best had in the period immediately following the discovery of insulin. In addition to his involvement in the commercial production of insulin, the social aspects of the landmark event had a profound effect on the life of young Charles Best. In other words, to the young Charlie Best, the worldwide publicity and the adulation heaped upon the discoverers felt like all his Christmases had come at once.

Patents for Insulin

In 1922 the Canadian, US and British patent offices granted a patent for insulin in the names of Banting, Best and Collip. The three men immediately assigned the patents to the University of Toronto Board of Governors, thus ensuring that no commercial interests would be in a position to exploit patients. The board was empowered to oversee the granting of licenses to manufacturers with a stipulation that 50% of the profits be given to the University for research and the rest to Banting, Best and Collip for their scientific work.

Canada's insulin was supplied by the Connaught Laboratories which were owned by the University of Toronto. The company later developed into a major pharmaceutical firm and became one of the largest drug manufacturing concerns in Canada.

In 1972 the Connaught Laboratories were sold by the University of Toronto to the Canada Development Corporation. The proceeds from the sale, $24 million, were placed in a special fund at the Toronto University to support its research projects. Charles Best, who that time was a Professor of Physiology at university, was put in charge of the fund. The following story may interest students of medical history.

The Professor and a Curious Story of Money Laundering–for a Good Cause

The University of Toronto continued to collect royalties from the sale of insulin in the United States and Canada. Between 1923 and 1967, this resulted in an income of some 8 million for the University.

The indefatigable Michael Bliss managed to unearth a case of possible "money-laundering" from this fund. It is included here because of the prominence of at least two of the central characters in the insulin story.

Oskar Minkowski (1858–1931) whose central role in the pursuit of insulin has already been described, died in 1931. Born in a village in Russia, Minkowski was Jewish and adhered to his faith throughout his life much of which was spent in Germany. He was married to Marie Siegel who was still alive when the Second World War broke out in 1939. With the rising persecution of Jews she wanted to escape from Germany.

During the search for insulin, there had been close contact between the Toronto workers and Minkowski because of his prominence in the scientific world in general but especially because of his seminal observations on the role of the pancreas in the production of insulin.

The income from insulin royalties was kept apart from the other streams of income allocated to the university. Insulin royalties were meant to be used only for research. However, the records of the fund's expenditures in 1941 document a transfer of moneys with a cryptic one word description, "Minkowski". In actual fact the money was used to assist the escape of Minkowski's widow to South America.

The University's Research Fund was controlled by the then Professor of Physiology and Head of the Department, Charles Herbert Best.

Toronto's Generosity.
International Patents for Manufacture of insulin

In today's increasingly competitive world of commerce the generosity of the authorities responsible for the initial production of insulin in Toronto is almost beyond belief.

Firstly, the Toronto workers especially Banting never tried to keep their work a secret. Locally, that is in Toronto University, it was well known that experiments were being carried out "on Insulin". As has been repeatedly stated, Banting was entirely focussed on finding insulin and putting it to use in the treatment of patients as soon as practicable. That he had not been aware of the steps between the bench in the laboratory and the bedside of the stricken is clear. His own experience in the use of insulin on patients will be described later. What must be acknowledged is that the Insulin Committee of Toronto University unhesitatingly and generously made the details of the processes involved in making the insulin extract widely available.

After much discussion the University of Toronto filed a patent application on the discovery of insulin to cover both insulin it self as well as the methods of isolation and purification developed by the researchers in Toronto. The University established an

Insulin Committee* which was charged with the responsibility of administering "the patents in the public interest". Its intention was to use its industrial property rights for two purposes namely, to control and maintain the standard and quality of insulin and secondly to prevent the emergence of any commercial interests which might attempt to monopolise the market with the potential of disadvantaging patients with diabetes.

On our January 23, 1923 the American patent for manufacture of insulin was granted to Banting, Best and Collip for $1 each. They then sold the patent to the University of Toronto for one dollar each.

In the United States the first patent was granted to the Eli Lilly Company of Indianapolis in 1922. However in order to guard against a monopoly in the sale of insulin the University of Toronto granted patents to several small and large institutions in the United States in the second half of 1922 and in 1923.

Internationally Toronto University extended the patent to 25 countries in North America, Latin America, Britain, European countries, Australia, India and Japan. The early prominence of the Lilly Company in the manufacture of insulin had raised concerns in some quarters of the potential disadvantages mentioned above.

The question of the use of insulin "in the public interest" was only partly resolved by the patents being granted to the large number countries as noted above. This did not silence some critics who were opposed to the idea of royalties being collected by the

---

* The Insulin Committee was composed of three members from the Board of Governors of the University including Sir Robert Falconer, an advisory committee made up of the four researchers namely Frederick Banting, Charles Best, Bertram Collip and John J.R. Macleod and the director of Connaught Laboratories John Fitzgerald. The committee set up a Laboratory to check on the quality of insulin produced by different pharmaceutical firms. Later prominent physicians and researchers as well as members of the pharmaceutical industry were added to the committee. Charles Riches, a lawyer specialising in laws on patents was the first attorney appointed to the committee.

University of Toronto even though all monies received were to finance it's medical research.

Insulin was retained as the name of the product. It had been first suggested by J. deMeyer in 1909, then by Edward Schaffer in 1916.

The commonest brand name in the early years was Iletin used by the Eli Lilly Company.

The rapidity with which insulin from the laboratory was delivered to patients with diabetes was impressive, to say the least. Within 12 months of its discovery it was available to patients in Toronto and then in the following 12 months to patients in the United States and Britain. The Connaught Laboratories in Toronto and the Eli Lilly Company in Indianapolis were the earliest centres of manufacture. In Europe, through the Danish pharmaceutical company Nordisk insulin production had begun in 1923. In the early years of insulin production Eli Lilly's international arm was the major supplier to countries as far afield as Australia.

Some accounts of the introduction of Insulin especially in England and Europe provide interesting insights into the early history of insulin.

The Introduction of Insulin in England

The first mention of offering the patent for manufacturing insulin to Britain was in June 1922 when Macleod had written to the secretary of the medical research council (MRC) indicating the University of Toronto's offer to the MRC patent rights to the "anti-diabetic extract". The following month Fitzgerald travelled to England and discussed the situation with the officers of the Council. The MRC at that time was a young organisation which had been created by the British Government just before the First World War as a branch of the British health insurance industry. The MRC scientists were sceptical considering the new product insulin possibly being one of the host of miracle cures which were quite common and had little scientific basis. At that time to the very conservative scientists in the MRC this kind of overture was considered with strong reservations, even scepticism. It was from a little known University's medical school in one of "the colonies".

As noted earlier Dr Henry H. Dale, Director of the Biochemistry and Pharmacology Department of the council's National Institute for Medical Research suggested that he and a biochemist colleague, Harold Dudley, visit Toronto to look at the alleged discovery.

Even though Dale and Dudley confirmed the veracity of Toronto's claims, when eventually the MRC reluctantly accepted control of the British patent the prevailing view amongst the scientific fraternity in Britain was that a patent was unnecessary. There was only grudging admission of it's possible advantages.

It is a fact of history that on May 16, 1923, insulin became commercially available in Great Britain, the first country to provide the extract from its pharmacies to diabetics, physicians and hospitals.

The reason for Britain receiving such preferred treatment becomes clearer when viewed in the context of that period in the history of Canada in general and Toronto in particular.

In 1921 Toronto had a population of around half a million. Between 30 and 40% of the population had been born in the United Kingdom. Its inhabitants were largely working-class and toiled for long hours for low wages in factories and concerns like the Gooderham and Worts distillery. Inner-city districts like Cabbage Town were dotted with rundown dwellings which afforded accommodation to the largely English and Irish colonial immigrants and their descendants. Toronto's first large hotel, the Casa Loma opened in 1927 renting rooms for six dollars a day. Its first Street Car (the Peter Witt) had started in October 1921. To most Torontonians around the time of the discovery of insulin England was very much "mother England."

Those in authority in England including Dale harboured reservations if not scepticism towards the discovery. Thus clinical testing in Britain did not begin till the end of the year. In the meantime in America hundreds of lives had been saved and the condition of the starved and wasted diabetics dramatically improved by the use of insulin.

Dale had emphasised the importance of carrying out experiments to confirm the effectiveness of insulin manufactured on a large scale.

Tragically, fewer than 50 diabetics in eight different centres in Britain had received insulin by the end of 1922 and early 1923.

A tragic postscript to Paula Ing's diabetes was that she only received insulin in March 1923 but, either from the quality or the quantity of the insulin given, she lapsed into coma and died in March 1923.

As had happened in Toronto, the medical teams in England which were assigned the task of producing insulin were no match for the industrial behemoth Lilly. By the end of March 1923 Lilly was offering to supply insulin to the English. Fortunately, common sense won out and the commercial interests of British manufacturers including Burroughs Wellcome, Allen and Hanburys and British Drug Houses had to take second-place to the needs of the patients many of whom were dying because of the lack of Insulin.

Large supplies of insulin manufactured by Lilly arrived promptly to save the day for hundreds of British patients.

Insulin Manufacture in Europe

One of the earliest European countries to begin manufacturing insulin was Denmark.

A letter dated October 23, 1922 from the Danish chemist and Nobel laureate August Krogh to James Macleod gratefully acknowledges the authorisation from the Torontonians to start work in Denmark on the extract developed in Toronto. Krogh together with Hans Christian Hagedorn started the Nordisk Insulin laboratorium which went on to become one of the more prominent suppliers of insulin initially in Europe but later, as an internationally prominent pharmaceutical company, throughout the world.

The background of this Danish insulin company provides a fascinating insight into the history of pharmacy in Denmark.

More than 400 years earlier, on 12 September, 1620, the Danish king Christian IV awarded the Lion Pharmacy Royal license to manufacture and sell pharmaceutical products. Even in those early times there was clear recognition of the need for full control over those who were entrusted with the manufacture and sale of pharmaceutical products. The Lion Pharmacy had survived the great fires which had ravaged Copenhagen in 1728 and 1795. Aware and respectful of its history, Kongsted and Peterson were determined to continue, indeed enhance the standing of the firm in the commercial landscape not only of Scandinavia but the entire continent of Europe. They established a laboratory in the basement of the pharmacy soon after its acquisition. There were only three members on the staff of the new firm.

In 1908 August Kongsted and Anton Peterson bought the Leo pharmacy situated on the main shopping street of Copenhagen.

It was August Kongsted who provided Krogh and Hagedorn with the financial assistance needed by them to get their pharmaceutical company started. However Kongsted had stipulated that the fledgeling company's insulin be named Leo, the Latin word for lion.

Both Krogh and Hagedorn embarked on a period of intensive research conducting experiments to develop an effective extract of insulin. Hagedorn worked in his laboratory at home and Krogh in the Laboratory of Zoo-physiology at the Krogh Institute.

The reader will undoubtedly have noticed the difference in the academic and scientific backgrounds of the two men compared with Banting and Best. Krogh was a Nobel laureate and Hagedorn a qualified chemist experienced in preparing solutions and extracts. Little wonder then that on 21 December, 1922 they succeeded in producing a small batch of insulin from bovine pancreas. Unlike the difficulties in obtaining supplies of bovine pancreas in Toronto, the pancreas of slaughtered pigs was in abundant supply in Denmark because of the fondness of the Danes for bacon. Krogh was so thrilled by their success in isolating insulin that 10 days later, 2nd January, 1923 he set aside his laboratory work on the physiology of circulation to concentrate on insulin. It is not uncommon for men and women engaged in complex scientific studies which require long hours of what can be tedious laboratory work to be attracted to a "practical" project and the potential of insulin in the treatment of diabetes would understandably have attracted Krogh. Whether he was prepared for what was to follow next is another matter!

The first insulin marketed in Scandinavia in the spring of 1923 was insulin Leo. The following year when the company was organised as an independent concern, Kongsted joined Hagedorn and Krogh as part of the management team.

To build the machinery needed in the manufacturing plant, Krogh and Hagedorn employed Harald Pedersen. Pedersen was known for his inventive capabilities and found the challenge of building the required machinery attractive and well within his capabilities.

Pedersen remained with the insulin producing company for several years but the association ended soon after Pedersen's brother Thorvald, a pharmacist hired by Nordisk to conduct analysis of insulin solutions clashed with Hagedorn. In April 1924 Hagedorn fired Thorvald Pederson. To maintain family solidarity his brother Harald left with him.

Exceptionally hard-working and expert in their fields the two brothers, within months of starting their newly formed Novo Company produced a stable insulin extract which was released in the spring of 1924.

Harald Pedersen also designed the Novo syringe which simplified drawing up the correct dose of insulin into the syringe and injecting it. The needle was much finer and went a long way to overcoming another troublesome aspect of treating diabetes, namely the pain of injecting.

At first the brothers wanted to work with all this because neither of them was confident of running a commercial operation. Hagedorn however neither forgot nor forgave easily. He flatly rejected all overtures of conciliation and corporation. As for August Krogh the dedicated laboratory scientist, the hard-nosed approach of Hagedorn on commercial matters was entirely foreign to him. So he stayed out of all the acrimonious commercial negotiations.

In contrast with the production of insulin in America where Lilly dominated the market, Denmark had two successful companies producing insulin. Novo quickly established overseas markets and became a major supplier of Insulin around the world.

The novo syringe was the forerunner of a host of innovations aimed at firstly, reducing mistakes in drawing up the correct amount of insulin and secondly, addressing the problem of portability of insulin syringes and the discomfort associated with injecting insulin.

Eventually the two Danish companies merged to form today's Novo Nordisk Company.

In Germany the patent was granted to Febwerk Hoechst in 1923.

Clinical trials of Insulin

On November 25 1922, doctors prominent in the treatment of diabetes met in Toronto to discuss the clinical use of insulin. The meeting was held in the library of the medical building at the University of Toronto.

17 doctors were present. It is interesting to note the very marked disparity in knowledge and experience in treating diabetes between the Torontonians in that group and the invited Americans.

Gilchrist and Banting who were treating diabetics in the Christie Street Clinic had never treated patients with diabetes before then. Gilchrist, himself a diabetic had been treated with a restricted diet before starting Insulin a few months earlier. Banting had only seen one patient with diabetes before starting on the experiments leading to the discovery of insulin. He had no practical experience in treating diabetics with a restricted diet. He had negligible experience in the use of insulin in human subjects. Fletcher and Campbell had become involved with the treatment of diabetic patients at the Toronto General Hospital but had little practical knowledge. Toronto General did not have a Diabetic Clinic. Duncan Graham will no doubt have invited himself as the Head of the Department of Medicine.

The group from America included Elliott Joslin from Boston, Rollin Woodyatt from Chicago, John Williams and Russell Wilder from Rochester, Frederick Allen and Rawle Graylin from New York, Arthur Walters and John McDonald from Indianapolis, and J.H.A. Clowse from Lilly. Anton Carlson had sent his apologies.

The physicians from the United States, who outnumbered the Torontonians, were far more knowledgeable. Many, like Woodyatt and Allen had been engaged in research on the condition and treating diabetic children and adults for years. Joslin who had a register for each diabetic patient seen in his practice had documented detailed information in a register of some 3000 diabetics at that time. His textbook based on this number was released in 1923 shortly after the announcement of the discovery of insulin.

Most of the clinical trials of insulin developed in Toronto were carried out by physicians in America including Joslin, Allen and Woodyatt.

Six months later the results of the trials carried out on diabetics treated with insulin were published in the November – December 1923 issue of the *Journal of Metabolic Research*. This scientific periodical had been started by Francis Allen who was its editor.

However, as early as February 1923, Insulin usage had become widespread especially in Canada and United States where over 1000 patients in 60 clinics supervised by around 250 physicians were receiving the hormone. By the end of the year the number of patients receiving insulin had increased to over 25,000 in the United States alone.

Arrangements for producing insulin rapidly spread to other countries.

PART FOUR
INSULIN CELEBRATED

CANADA'S FIRST NOBEL PRIZE

As soon as the discovery of insulin was announced, there was effusive recognition for Banting at home and beyond. Everyone wanted to see him, hear him speak, reward him and add his name to their organisation regardless of the absence of any previous acquaintances or association.

The celebrations took various forms beginning at the end of December, 1922 at the Toronto meeting of the Federation of American Societies for Experimental Biology where he received a standing ovation. Members of the New York Academy of medicine cheered him as soon as he arrived at the meeting as a guest speaker. In the nation's capital Ottawa, at a banquet held in his honour, the Canadian Prime Minister and Leader of the Opposition spoke of him in glowing terms.

Crowds lined the streets to give him a hero's welcome when he came to his hometown of Alliston where his parents still lived on their dairy farm.

The business community embraced him as a national hero with honorary membership to the exclusive clubs. He became the favourite guest speaker at luncheons.

In the summer of 1923 Banting was invited to England and Europe as a guest lecturer to speak at medical and scientific conferences. The fact that his limitations in public speaking were well known within medical circles did not diminish the ardour of the organisers of such medical meetings.

In England he was honoured by a special audience with King George V.

Banting was invited to open the Canadian National Exhibition, probably the first physician to be so honoured by the national institution which dates its beginnings to 1879.

Although primarily an agricultural exhibit, in later years it also included innovations. However insulin had displaced all other innovations and discoveries at this time.

At the urging of some of Banting's friends some Toronto newspapers started a campaign for Banting to be awarded the Nobel Prize but after a few months the momentum slowed to a halt.

In May 1923 the Ontario government announced that the University of Toronto was establishing the Banting and Best Chair of Medical Research, a non-teaching professorship to Banting, and a grant of $10,000 to pay for Banting's salary, support research and fund Best's research. A special appropriation of $10,000 was given to Banting to reward him for his discovery. According to Michael Bliss, Banting gave $2,500 of this grant to Best.

On August 27, 1923 Banting was featured on the cover of Time magazine, the first Canadian to be so honoured.

Postage stamps featuring Banting have appeared regularly since 1923.

In 1934 he was made a Knight of the British Empire (KBE), thereby becoming Sir Frederick Banting. It is said that he did not like the title but others especially in the United States regarded it as a great honour. The Boston diabetes specialist Elliott Joslin, who devoted a chapter in his instruction manual for patients to insulin, included a black-and-white photograph of Banting in academic dress and from 1934 on never failed to refer to him as Sir Frederick Banting in his manuals and textbooks. The Americans may have resented being the subjects of the British kings and queens but never lost their interest in, or fascination with, English titles. In Canada there appears to be ambivalence towards English honours but one suspects that some still cherish the hope of getting one. Charles Best kept up his contact with his British colleagues throughout his life and according to his family records, cherished his contact with British royalty.

Even though he had the appointment and facilities for research, Banting never really returned to serious research work. Perhaps this was well known to those who advised those who gifted the Nobel Laureate with an academic appointment at Toronto University that the appointment to be specified as "non-teaching" in order to free him from any regular commitment not only to students but also to younger researchers. In fact the position was simply yet another form of rewarding him.

The Banting Institute for Medical Research was initially separate from a similar institution for Charles Best but was later combined into The Banting and Best Institute for Medical Research.

The Nobel Prize for Physiology or Medicine 1923

Toronto etched its name in the annals of medical history on October 23, 1923 when the Nobel Prize for Physiology or Medicine was awarded to Banting and Macleod.

The crowning glory for the discovery of insulin was undoubtably winning the Nobel Prize for Physiology or Medicine in 1923. Banting, who won the prize with the unanimous approval of the members of the Nobel Committee remains the youngest winner of the prize in that division to this day. He was also the first Canadian to win the award. Perhaps his putting Canada "on the map" and in such prestigious company makes the effusive outpouring of national pride and gratitude through the many titles, gifts and honours understandable, even justified.

In the insulin story, 1923 will be remembered mainly for the first Nobel prize to be awarded to a Canadian for its discovery.

News of the award reached Toronto by a telegram carried by the Canadian Pacific Railway Company sent from Stockholm dated October 25. It read as follows:

DOCTOR FREDERICK G BANTING
INSTITUTE OF PHYSIOLOGY
TORONTO CANADA
THE ROYAL CAROLINE INSTITUTE HAS PRESENTED
  TO YOU TOGETHER WITH PROFESSOR WJR
  MACLEOD THE NOBEL PRIZE OF THE YEAR 1923.
YOURS SINCERELY HJALMAR FORSSNER PRINCIPAL
  OF THE INSTITUTE
10.30 PM.

Established in 1901 from the estate of the Swedish industrialist Alfred Bernhard Nobel (1833–1896), the Nobel Prize is generally regarded as the most prestigious award in the different fields it covers. According to Nobel's will the prize was intended for a discovery in medicine or physiology which "conferred the greatest benefit on mankind."

The committee responsible for deciding the recipient/s of the prize has its set of rules. It is not bound by any conditions which would require it to state its reasons for deciding on the winner/s. Its decision is final. It does not engage in any discussion especially relating to the whys and wherefores apart from that which is stated at the time of announcing the winners.

Nobel Prize 1923 a New Star In The Galaxy Of Science

"Go to hell."
    Banting's Initial reaction to winning the Nobel Prize

October 26,1923 was a Friday. Banting had spent the previous night visiting his parents in Alliston. When he entered his office the phone was ringing. It was Jerry Fitzgerald.

"Congratulations, have you seen the papers?"

Banting said he had not.

"You and Macleod got the Nobel prize," said Fitzgerald.

"Go to hell," said Canada's first Nobel Prize winner. Presumably he had not received the telegram sent through the Canadian Pacific Railway Company's Telegraph service.

Bliss's book contains a dramatic account of Banting being angry at Macleod's inclusion in the award which would not have surprised any of those associated with the project given the strained relations between the two men was common knowledge. The essence of Banting's objection to Macleod's inclusion was that the latter had not made any significant contribution to the project. In fact Macleod had been in Scotland for his annual summer holidays when the two researchers had isolated an extract and shown it to be effective. Banting was also distressed that his student helper Charles Best had not been recognised by the Nobel Committee.

Bliss's colourful description of Banting's tirade was related to me more than once. However I was unable to find any reference in his notes on the source of his version of the incident.

Fitzgerald, obviously delighted with Banting's award was waiting for him on the steps to the building which housed Fitzgerald's office as well as the Department of Physiology where Banting was headed. Fitzgerald calmed Banting down and told him that Colonel Gooderham, a prominent member of the Board of Governors of the University of Toronto, was waiting for him in his university office.

The philanthropist was one man whom Banting respected. Gooderham, for his part, respected the decorated soldier. The whiskey magnate was himself a Civil War veteran. Gooderham listened patiently to Banting's reaction to the prize. He then reminded the Nobel laureate of the glory the prize would bring not only to Banting but to all of Canada and to every Canadian. He stressed the importance of putting Canada first.

Then, as was typical of the philanthropist, he told Banting to "catch the first boat to Stockholm" to receive the prize in person and asked him to stop by his office to collect the funds necessary for the journey as a personal gift from him to Canada's first Nobel Laureate. He reminded the now somewhat calmer Banting that he did not want him to be remembered as being the first Canadian to receive the honour only to reject it. Sensing that he was gaining ground, Gooderham stressed the importance of the respect the world had for scientists chosen as being worthy of receiving the Nobel Prize. Finally, he asked Banting to consider what the scientific fraternity around the world would think of one of their number rejecting the prize on the basis of his own opinion. He suggested that Banting reflect on these matters and wait for at least 24 hours before making his own final decision.

Banting, for once, heeded the advice and decided there and then to share the prize – and the credit.

Fitzgerald's people-skills and Gooderham's fatherly counsel had salvaged the situation and avoided a potentially regrettable and embarrassing incident for the university, Toronto, and Canada as a whole. That they were not going to change Banting's opinion of Macleod is part of the history of the discovery of insulin.

It is clear from several accounts that winning the Nobel Prize had not been prominent in Banting's thinking. However, the possibility had been raised with him by at least one medical acquaintance. During the early stages of finding practicable ways of producing insulin on a large scale, the Lilly director of research Clowse had suggested to Banting a plan for publishing an article on the method of testing the batches of insulin produced in different centres including Toronto, before Indianapolis, and recently, the smaller facilities in America like the one headed by Woodyatt in Chicago. Clowse told Banting that the article could be published in a special issue of Frederick Allen's *Journal of Metabolic Research* with Banting as the lead author. Clowse then went even further in suggesting something which may have been frowned on by the scientific fraternity of the time as it would be today. He told the young researcher that the Lilly Company would underwrite the expenses of the distribution of Banting's article throughout the US.

Bliss in his book quoted a letter from Clowse to Banting dated 11th of August 1922 stating "and if this were done, you would not only get full credit for your work but it would be the first step towards receiving the Nobel Prize in medicine for you and your associates."

Given Banting's insecurities over the issue of priority in his research on isolating insulin, it is unlikely that he would have warmed to Clowse's suggestion of the prize being shared with his associates especially if the group included Macleod. That this not only turned out to be true but ironically, largely because of Banting, took centre stage, will be described later. It is clear however, that Banting at that time was entirely focussed on the problem of getting insulin to those who need it most, namely the patients. It is doubtful if he had given the possibility of winning the Nobel prize much thought. After all, no one in Canada had ever won the prize coveted by many if not most scientists. Canada, especially Toronto, was hardly ever considered prominent as a centre of medical research. They certainly were not in the same league as the traditional long-established universities with their associated research laboratories in France, Germany, Britain, and in later years, the United States.

Frederick Banting's Nobel Lecture. September 15, 1925

Banting began his Nobel lecture with the story of von Merring and Minkowski producing severe diabetes when they removed the pancreas of dogs. The dogs invariably died. This had revealed the pancreas as the organ which harbours "an internal secretion". Banting had reasoned that diabetes could perhaps be treated with an extract of the pancreas containing this hitherto elusive secretion. Treatment with many different extracts had, up to that time, achieved only temporary success. He cited the work of several scientists including Scott and Paulesco who had obtained extracts from the pancreas which had produced positive results.

Highlighting recent advances, and for the purposes of his work, especially timely were the methods which, for the first time, had enabled investigators to measure the amount of glucose present in small volumes of blood much more quickly than they had been able to with previous older methods. Banting paid tribute to pioneers in this field naming Benedict, Folin and Wu. Also at the same time, there was an increasing awareness of the importance of different classes of food – proteins, carbohydrates and fat. In this context Banting mentioned the highly respected German diabetes specialist Carl von Noorden, and the prominent Americans, Frederick Allen, Elliott Joslin, and Rollin Woodyatt, All these men, especially Elliott Joslin, had encouraged, helped and supported Banting in his work after their initial meeting at the American Society of Physiologists conference at Yale – Banting had never forgotten that. He and Best had met Joslin frequently and there had been regular correspondence with him. Handwritten letters from both Banting and Best attest to the Boston physician's relationship with the two young Canadians. The archives at the Joslin Diabetes Centre afforded me the privilege of examining these and later provided copies of handwritten correspondence between the two researchers and Joslin. He remained a mentor to Banting and especially to Best for the rest of their lives.

Banting spoke of the germ of the idea in the early hours of the morning when he had trouble going to sleep. It would not have been appropriate for him to mention that it was also the time when his fiancé Edith Roach had broken her engagement to him. Neither would the coincidence of Halloween with his flash of insight been appropriate to be shared with the august audience which included royalty and the cream of European scientific aristocracy.

Banting recounted the beginning of the journey on April 14, 1921 in the "physiological laboratory of the University of Toronto where Professor Macleod allotted me Dr Charles Best." He went on to describe the different extracts which had been used and gave details of the methods of making the extract. Relating the beneficial effect on three patients in Toronto General Hospital he did not omit the complication of formation of painful abscesses at the site of the injections.

Following the sequence of events related above, Banting noted that it was February 1922 (10 months after he and Best had started) when "Professor Macleod abandoned his work on anoxaemia and turned his whole laboratory staff on to the investigation of the physiological properties of what is now known as insulin."

Collip's contribution was noted as was the role of Best in taking over the large–scale production of insulin at the Connaught Laboratories under the guidance of Professor Fitzgerald "who is kind enough to be here today."

(What wealth of recollections was in the new Nobel Laureate's heart and mind in that brief reference to the incomparable Fitzgerald. It was Fitzgerald who had sensed Banting's dedication to his work as well as his shortcomings, especially in public relations, from the first time he had met the aspiring scientist in April 1921.)

Banting then proceeded to describe the use of insulin on patients in the recently established diabetic clinics of Toronto General Hospital as well as in The Hospital for Sick Children. He emphasised the difference between those treated with diet alone versus those in whom insulin had been added to the treatment program.

Reading through the lecture it becomes clear that Banting was selfless and generous when it came to the help he had received in his pursuit of insulin.

The largest part of his lecture when acknowledging help from others was devoted to the guidance of Elliott Joslin of Boston.

In closing, perhaps as a gentle rebuke to those who had been quick to leap to the conclusion that insulin was a "miracle cure" for diabetes, Banting emphasised that "insulin is not a cure for diabetes; it is a treatment."

His closing remarks were a simple summary which were for the benefit of the lay members in the audience. He told them that insulin could be used "to provide energy for coping with the economic burdens of life."

The applause was thunderous. Many stood. Those seated close to the lectern will not have failed to see the look of relief on Banting's face. He had never sought the limelight. He was never comfortable in it and had tried to avoid it even after the constant companionship of fame following the worldwide recognition of the importance of the discovery of insulin.

AFTER THE GLORY

THE LATER LIFE OF
FREDERICK BANTING

Banting's fame from the discovery of insulin did not diminish with time. He continued to be deluged with requests to give lectures, open new buildings, often not related to insulin in any way whatsoever. People simply wanted him for his reputation derived from the achievement which has guaranteed him a permanent place in history.

Numerous schools, parks, public buildings and other institutions have been named after him. The Banting House at the national historic site of Canada has given him an enduring visibility in the nation's history. The house purchased by the Canadian Diabetic Association in 1981 is preserved as a museum to celebrate not only to a great Canadian discovery but also the life and medical research of Sir Frederick Grant Banting. The Association has recreated his office in the original bedroom. Its offices are confined to the back of the building.

A visit to Banting House is on the itinerary of most visiting dignitaries. In 1989 her Majesty Queen Elizabeth the Queen Mother visited Banting House to unveil the bronze statue of Banting writing down his insulin hypothesis. She also kindled the Flame of Hope which will burn until a cure for diabetes is found on which occasion the discover/s of the cure will be brought to

London, Ontario to extinguish the flame and unearth the time capsule buried in 1991 as part of the celebrations of the centenary of Banting's birth.

After his work on insulin, Banting's attempts at scientific exercise in the laboratory yielded little if any constructive results. He is said to have developed an interest in painting and demonstrated some talent.

What persisted and has received less interest than deserved is the human side of Banting especially in his treatment of patients. Several such incidents have been described already; his bedside vigil and treatment throughout the night of James Havens, and his compassion for his friend and his first patient Joe Gilchrist.

Bliss recounted the story of Leonard Thompson who had been rescued from death by insulin. Thompson whose diabetes had been diagnosed in 1919 had been kept alive on a restricted diet for two years but was all skin and bone in 1921.

The first injection on January 11, 1921 of the extract prepared by Best had failed. Then at 11 am on Monday, January 23, 1921 Thompson had been injected with the improved extract prepared by Collip. That history-making injection of insulin proved to be "the medical shot heard round the world."

Thompson had a second relapse when the initial batch of Collip's extract had run out and the researcher was unable to reproduce the method by which he had made the first successful extract. As a result Thompson, together with several other patients who had been started on insulin was discharged without a supply of insulin. They had to manage without it for at least six weeks and were all in dire straits until once again they were all, including Thompson saved by insulin. This time the Insulin extracts had been prepared in the Connaught Laboratories under the supervision of Charles Best.

After starting back on three or four injections of insulin each day, Thompson had become accustomed to his new routine and regained his health and a sense of wellbeing. He had worked in a chemical factory for 14 years. He was injecting himself with 85 units of insulin each day. He had had one emergency admission to Toronto General in 1932 but had recovered.

His final illness was pneumonia after he had contracted influenza. His diabetes on this occasion had proved difficult to control and progressed to acidosis. On April 20, 1935 the 27-year-old died in Toronto General Hospital.

Insulin had given him 14 years of a comparatively normal life.

Another part of this story which has perhaps been overshadowed by personality clashes between Banting and Macleod in particular is equally important because it shows the human side of Fred Banting. His compassion for his patients as is seen in his conversation with the young medical resident medical officer at Toronto General Hospital who had carried out the autopsy on Thompson.

Banting had asked if "the poor boy had remained on a high fat, low carbohydrate diet all these years."

When the resident, who had also looked after Thompson said yes, Banting asked if he had stuck to his diet. Again the answer was yes.

Then the Nobel Laureate asked the question which typifies one who sees a patient as a human being complete with the faults and foibles common to all.

"Did he have any fun?"

"Yes he had some fun. He used to get drunk nearly every weekend," answered the resident medical officer.

"Well, I'm glad he had some fun."

Whatever the criticisms were of Banting, his concern for the patient always took precedence over other issues. The fact that this may not have been given as much prominence as perhaps deserved can be attributed to the fact that the two books mentioned here, which provided excellent and comprehensive accounts were written by men who were not doctors. At times doctors, perhaps rightly, are accused of treating the illness and not the person suffering from it. In the majority of cases however, although the physician may at times be seen to be concentrating on the illness more than on the person is, in my opinion, a misconception in the vast majority of cases. It is more often a consequence of poor communication by the doctor – and here I include myself ahead of any of my colleagues – more than poor management of the patient.

In later years Banting is said to have developed a serious interest in oil painting and is said to have produced some creditable works.

His private life never achieved the stability and bliss of his younger colleague Charles Best. Banting, clearly still in love with Edith Roach tried in vain to re-establish their friendship but did not succeed and their relationship ended in 1924. Shortly afterwards Banting, still basking in the glory of the Nobel prize, married a socially prominent Marian Robertson, a doctor's daughter. They had met when Robertson was an x-ray technician at Toronto General Hospital during the time of the discovery of insulin. They had a son, William in 1929. Unfortunately the marriage did not last and they divorced in 1932.

In 1939 Banting married Henrietta Ball. She had worked as a laboratory technician in his department at the University of Toronto. Later she had become his research assistant. They did not have any children. Lady Banting later went to medical school and after graduating did research work on treatments for cancer. She attended functions held in honour of her husband. Banting's earlier associations with various institutions were revived when he became famous and Lady Banting was always available to speak at such functions. For example when Sir Frederick Banting Secondary School was opened in London (from where, you will recall, he could not wait to get away because he had not been able to gather enough patients to establish a viable medical practice), Lady Banting was there to give a speech. In 1970 she unveiled a plaque at Banting House to declare it a *London Public Library Historic Site.*

Approaching middle life, Banting was less inclined to lose his temper. He overcame his dislike and distrust of Collip. His association with Best diminished. Banting's fame and prominence in Canada may have had something to do with this though Best moving to England after his graduation as suggested by Sir Henry Dale may have also contributed to gradual cooling of their relationship. The English physiologist who had won the Nobel Prize for physiology or medicine in 1936 had become a mentor to Best even before the latter had completed medical school in Toronto. Dale was obviously taken by the young medical student involved in the discovery of insulin during his visit to Toronto in 1922.

Just as the First World War had played a significant role in Frederick Banting's life, so as it turned out, did the Second World War which began in 1939. Predictably, given his prominence, Banting's attempt to enlist as an Army Medical Officer was rejected. He was persuaded to accept a more senior and responsible position which involved chairing a medical research committee working on Canada's war time activities. He spent the winter of 1939 and 1940 in London (England) working with his English counterparts.

According to Michael Bliss, Banting's writings on the discovery of insulin did not produce an account considered worthy of publication. He was inclined to be rambling and disorganised. As seen repeatedly during his pursuit of insulin, Banting had never been one to seek assistance or advice let alone guidance especially when he felt strongly about an issue or the way it was to be described.

Banting returned to Canada in 1940.

On February 20, 1941 he boarded a Hudson bomber in Gander, Newfoundland bound for England. The reason for this journey is unclear. It had been a severe winter and the night of the takeoff was bitterly cold. Shortly after take-off the aircraft stalled apparently due to the formation of ice in a part of the engine. The plane crashed. Banting was rescued and transferred to hospital but but died shortly afterwards. He was 49.

Frederick Grant Banting, the son of a dairy farmer and the discoverer of insulin is buried in Mount Pleasant Cemetery in Toronto.

For his discovery Banting was awarded the Nobel Prize for Physiology or Medicine. He remains its youngest winner in that category.

Even though 100 years have passed since the event, his is the first name on everyone's lips when remembering the discovery which continues to relieve the suffering of millions every day.

Therein lies his glory.

The Co-recipient of the 1923 Nobel Prize for Physiology or Medicine James Macleod

Much has been written about the controversy over Macleod receiving a share of the Nobel Prize for the discovery of insulin. He was the head of the department in which the work was carried out and as such in common with many if not most institutions even today he would be ascribed due recognition. Whether that entitled him to receiving part of the award has been and remains an issue over which there has been considerable disagreement. This was largely fuelled by Frederick Banting himself whose role in the discovery of insulin was never questioned – neither at the time of the discovery nor when he was the awarded the Nobel Prize. Much of the publicity especially in Toronto can be attributed to the difficult relationship which existed between Banting and Macleod. Unfortunately, in spite of attempts by several members of the staff at the University of Toronto and Toronto General Hospital, the two men were never able to reconcile their differences. This aspect of the insulin story was seized upon particularly by Bliss and given considerable coverage in his book. The issue also featured prominently in the Best family papers but for a different reason as related in Henry Best's book when discussing Charles Best's role in the experiments carried out during the search for insulin.

The Best family papers contain considerable information on the visit of two Nobel laureates to Toronto. Both had been invited to Toronto and entertained as houseguests by Macleod who arranged lectures and dinners for them. Whether or not either of these men actively promoted the awarding of the Nobel Prize to James Macleod has remained a matter of speculation.

James Macleod's Nobel Lecture May 26, 1925

This is based on the material published online by the Nobel Foundation.

The work conducted in his department by Banting and Best occupied one of 27 paragraphs and appeared after a lengthy preamble.

Then the essence of the insulin project as conceived by Banting was covered in one sentence in which he included himself with Banting and Best.

"Believing that the want of success to prepare extracts of uniform potency as due to the destruction of the antidiabetic hormone by the digestive enzymes also present in the gland, F.G. Banting suggested preparing them from duct–ligated pancreas, and with the aid of C.H. Best, and under my direction, he succeeded in 1922 in showing that such extracts reduce the hyperglycaemia and glycosuria in depancreatised dogs."

The general symptoms of diabetes were also found to be alleviated and the duration of life of the depancreatised animal prolonged, by repeated injections of alcoholic extract of foetal, as well as adult ox pancreas. Later it was shown, in collaboration with Collip, that other symptoms of diabetes, namely ketonuria and the absence of glycogen from the liver were favourably influenced by the extract and, with Hepburn, that the respiratory quotient became raised. These results in depancreatised dogs showed beyond doubt that the antidiabetic hormone was present in potent form in the extracts, and the time seemed right to investigate their action on the clinical forms of diabetes. This was done by Banting in a severe case under the care of W.R. Campbell, with the result that the hyperglycaemia and glycosuria were diminished. At the same time, however, it was found that it would be necessary to rid the extract of irritating substances before the value of their repeated injection in the treatment of diabetes in man could be adequately put to the test. This was accomplished by Collip, and the name insulin was decided upon for the purified extract. This name had previously been suggested by Sir E. Sharpey Schafer (1916), who had been one of the first to support the hypothesis of the insular derivation of the antidiabetic hormone. I need not here detail the rapid progress which it was now possible to make in studying the therapeutic value of insulin in the treatment of diabetes in man; for it is with experimental aspects of the subject that this essay is concerned."

At no stage was there any mention of Banting succeeding where others, whom he had named, including E.L. Scott and Nicolae Paulescu, had failed. Nor did he mention the critical fact that only Banting was a qualified physician in the research team in Toronto to whom the use of insulin in human patients was an urgent priority. He was the only one who had actually been in medical practice.

Given that Banting had been the lone figure in the pursuit of insulin until its effect had been demonstrated in the experimental animal as presented in the meeting in New Haven, would it not have been reasonable or gracious of the Head of the Department to at least mention that to the august company? The lecture includes a detailed summary of previous work done in the search for insulin. Clearly, Banting and Best, who had spent the first part of the summer of 1920 studying the literature, had little if any knowledge of the background of investigations on insulin. Yet Macleod mentioned workers including Scott and Paulesco in his lecture. It is interesting that Macleod had given Charles Best as the topic for his final dissertation, "The Role of Pancreatic Extracts in the Utilisation of Carbohydrates by Diabetic Animals." This had been prepared and submitted to the university in the spring of 1922. Thus Macleod had detailed information on the work done by the two researchers in his department. As mentioned elsewhere in this work this particular document although filed in the Physiology Department of the University of Toronto and with "another university" has disappeared.

In the aftermath of the announcement of the discovery a reporter had asked Macleod what his role had been. Macleod laughed then made a facetious comment that he considered himself an "impresario." Perhaps the spontaneous reply was closer to the truth than the speaker had intended.

It is said that Macleod was shy and inclined to keep to himself. This may explain his reticence on occasions when he could have been more generous. Otherwise one can perhaps understand the frustrations, even anger on the part of Banting and later, also Charles Best at what appears to have been the absence of the virtues of grace and generosity on the part of the Head of the department where insulin was discovered.

Nobel Prize Controversies

Much has been written about the inclusion of Macleod and the exclusion of Best from the prize.

The enthusiasm for emphasising personal points of view often ignored the Nobel Committee's clearly stated criteria for awarding the prize as noted above. Clearly Bliss had found this to be a challenge, but also amusing when he had tried to obtain information from some of the people in Toronto who were "close to the action". He wrote:

"Well into the 1950s the oral history of the discovery of insulin was more interesting than the written history. There was a kind of underground of gossip, centring in Toronto medical circles and usually becoming more interesting after each round of drinks. Everybody who had been on the spot in 1921 and 1922 – professors in the university, medical students, residents and nurses in the hospital, friends of those involved – had stories to tell about what had *really* happened in those days, what the discoverers were really like, what their fights had been really about. The best stories were the ones that the discoverers themselves told. Banting, who died in 1941, and Best, who lived until 1978, tended to be the most talkative. J.J.R Macleod, who left Toronto in 1928 and died in 1935, had let slip an occasional bitter remark. J.B. Collip, who was never employed in Toronto after 1922 was a very discreet professor at McGill University and then Dean of Medicine at the

University of Western Ontario before his death in 1965. But even Collip would sometimes get talking about the insulin days. For all of them, after all, it was the greatest event of their lives."

Charles Best's Long Memory

It is interesting to record the comments of Charles Best's son Henry Best, the author of the book *Margaret and Charlie.*

Henry Best wrote that "the process of awarding the prize failed to operate properly in 1923 and is most responsible for the unfortunate result that has embarrassed the Nobel Committee ever since."

He noted the visit of August Krogh to Toronto from 23 to 25 November, 1922 when he was the house guest of the Macleod's for three days. Henry Best wrote that the three days would have allowed Macleod to emphasise his own role in the discovery of insulin. He also noted that Krogh was one of the few people allowed to make nominations for the Nobel Prize of 1923. The records indicate that Krogh did indeed nominate Macleod, but also Banting, for the Nobel Prize.

Clearly the matter had not been allowed to rest in Charles Best's family, even 70 years after the event because in 1961 Henry Best conducted an interview with Professor Rolf Luft who was then the secretary of the Nobel Committee.

Luft wrote to Henry Best who quoted the respected scientist's response: "I can say that, with reservations, I think that it might have been fair to give the prize to Banting, Best and * Paulesco."

Having met Professor Luft on more than one occasion at meetings of the International Diabetic Federation of which he was the President between 1973 and 1979, I think he would have found it awkward to revisit the Nobel controversy so many years after the event. Luft, a highly respected scientist and a consummate

---

* Nicolas Paulesco, a Roumanian scientist had published his own experiments with a pancreatic extract in 1921 and felt that he had done so before the discovery by the Toronto workers.

medical diplomat was known for his tact and commonsense, traits which are evident in his response to Henry Best.

One piece of information of relevance in the insulin story as to why Best, considered by some to be worthy of a share of the award, did not receive the prize is, quite simply, that he was never nominated. In fact Charles Best did not receive a single nomination for the award.

Another issue which was contested at the time and remains part of the controversy is the inclusion of all four participants namely Banting, Best, Collip and Macleod. This would not have been possible because the statutes of the Nobel Foundation specify that the maximum number of recipients for dividing the award into equal shares be limited to 3.

About the only part of the insulin story which, quite rightly, has not attracted controversy is Banting receiving the Nobel Prize. Would any of the other three have been prepared to give up half of their share?

Banting shared with Macleod the monitory value of the award and received the medal and the certificate as part of his prize. True to his word as usual, he gave half of the money to Best. Henry Best's book contains a 1927 photograph of the house at 226 Rosedale Heights Drive, Toronto which was purchased by Best partly with the gift from Banting.

"It was a comfortable home, with plenty of space. They paid $12,000, $9000 of which was Charlies half of Fred Banting's share of the Nobel Prize money."

Unlike Best, Banting was nominated for and awarded the Nobel Prize without any controversy. There is a concise and lucid account which clearly sets out the reasons for one person's opinion for his nomination. This was the nomination by Francis Gano Benedict. Benedict, a highly regarded scientist was the head of the Boston-based Nutrition Laboratory of the Carnegie Institution of Washington from 1907 to 1937. Indeed, the Boston branch of the research establishment had been built in order to retain Benedict's scientific contributions in the United States with the hope of preventing him being lured away from America by one of the many prestigious research centres in Europe.

Benedict's recommendation contained in the records of the Medical Nobel Committee was as follows:

"The one man pre-eminent above all others who should be considered for this remarkable work on the isolation of a pancreatic extract that will reduce blood sugar and has made marvellous changes in the treatment of diabetes. My only question was, first, should any of Dr. Banting's colleagues or confreres be mentioned as having contributed anything near an equal share in these researchers? To this I find the answer is "No." Second, since there are a number of people in America working on the pancreatic extract, is there anyone else whose claim for priority is liable to be seriously considered by scientists as a whole? To this I can also answer "No." Under the circumstances, therefore, I feel very confident in naming Dr Banting, and trust that the committee will be able to secure all the information they desire with regard to his work."

Did Two European House Guests Help Macleod to Get a Share of the Nobel Prize?

Predictably the discovery of insulin attracted the notice of the medical and scientific world because of the long history of diabetes and the frustrating search for the hormone considered central to its cause, at least at that time.

The English duo of Dale and Dudley were quickly followed by Europeans. Two early visitors were Professor August Krogh from Copenhagen and Professor Robert Barany from Uppsala, Sweden.

Krogh, who had won the Nobel Prize in 1920 for his scientific discoveries which dealt with various aspects of the anatomy and physiology of capillaries, was invited by Yale University to deliver the Silliman Memorial Lectures in August 1922.

Krogh and his wife Marie had travelled by sea and arrived in New York on November 23, 1922. He had given an illustrated lecture on some of his experiments on circulation in capillaries (microcirculation).

Krogh's wife had diabetes. Before coming to Toronto, they had met Elliott Proctor Joslin who, on hearing of Krogh's wife's diabetes, had told her of the discovery of insulin in Toronto. Marie Krogh was also a medical doctor and it was at her urging that Krogh had written to Macleod about visiting Toronto. Macleod, according to Henry Best was "obviously elated by Krogh's visit" mentioning it in letters to England and the United States as the reason he could not attend to other matters. The Kroghs stayed at the Macleods at 45 Nanton Avenue for three days. According to Henry Best, presumably from information obtained by his father, Macleod and Krogh had discussed the possibility of the Nobel Prize for the discovery of insulin.

Papers from the records of the Nobel Committee reveal that Krogh did indeed nominate Macleod as well as Banting for the award.

How much detail Macleod provided to Krogh and details of the process of obtaining insulin from animal tissue is unclear but what is significant is that when he left Toronto Krogh had the authorisation from the University of Toronto to produce insulin.

The canny Dane lost little time. Together with his Danish associate Hans Christian Hagedorn he worked feverishly during the winter of 1922-23 and succeeded in producing marketable insulin by the end of 1923 as described elsewhere in this book.

Largely through the efforts of Krogh and Hagedorn, Denmark's Insulin Leo, joined the American Isletin produced by Lilly laboratories, and insulin from Britain as the most prominent brands of the hormone on the market by late 1923.

The Danish insulin produced from pork had the advantage over beef insulin when it was found to be less likely to produce local allergic reactions when injected into the skin of diabetics. It was also favoured by many patients in countries like India where beef insulin was shunned on religious and cultural grounds.

The second European guest was Professor Robert Barany who, at the end of December 1922, had been present at the meeting of the Federation of American Society for Experimental Biology when Best and Clark Noble had presented a paper on the effect of insulin in rabbits. Barany, from Uppsala, Sweden had won the 1914 Nobel Prize for Physiology or Medicine in 1914 for his work on the physiology of hearing. In the letter to Macleod on 3rd January 1923, Barany was replying to an invitation by the Professor for him and his wife to stay as the Macleod's house-guests during their visit to Toronto. In the letter Barany thanked Macleod for the invitation which he accepted. From the Best family papers, Henry Best quoted that Barany in his letter also said "I thought that this discovery of insulin is of such importance that it should be awarded the Nobel Prize."

However there is no record of Barany nominating anyone for the Nobel Prize for Medicine or Physiology 1923.

Macleod expressing an interest in being nominated for the award on the grounds of providing "direction" to Banting and Best as he stated on more than one occasion is understandable. The discovery of insulin was after all, a scientific accomplishment of worldwide significance. Anyone associated with any aspect of the pursuit would have wanted to be part of that event – and the glory.

Including the name of the Head of the department in publications from academic centres where the work has been carried out is in keeping with the practices and conventions followed in many universities and research centres.

Whether those conventions should extend to the Head of the department seeking a share of the Nobel Prize is the crux of the question.

The Later Life of James Macleod

Those who return have never left

In 1928 at the age of 52, Macleod returned to his native Scotland as the Regius Professor at the University of Aberdeen, his alma mater from where he had graduated in Medicine and gained a PhD in 1898.

Although for the most of his professional life he had worked in the United States and Canada, Macleod's heart had always been in Scotland to which he had returned every year for his summer holidays. Even the possibility of the discovery of insulin when related to him by Banting and Best could not persuade him to cut short his holidays.

Regius professorships are unique in the academic circles of the United Kingdom and Ireland. It would have been an especially prized appointment for Macleod given the first Regius professorship had been given to a professor at the University of Aberdeen where it had originated by order of the Scottish King James the Fourth in 1497.

Macleod never spoke about the discovery of insulin. He lived peacefully for seven years and died from complications of severe arthritis in 1935. He was 59 years old.

His last professional and academic gesture was to nominate Charles Best to be elected as a Fellow of the Royal Society, FRS, generally regarded as one of the highest academic honours in the English-speaking world

Macleod's replacement as Professor of Physiology in Toronto University was his student Charles Best. Best was 29 years old and had graduated in medicine from the University of Toronto only three years earlier in 1925.

Collip's Later Life

As noted earlier, at the end of World War I Collip, then aged 27, was awarded a Rockefeller Travelling Fellowship starting April 1921 when he travelled to the University of Toronto to work with James Macleod, largely because of the Scotsman's known expertise on carbohydrate metabolism. He was present at a meeting between Macleod and Banting and knew of

Banting's proposed project to prepare an extract of the pancreas with which to treat diabetes.

Collip joined the team in December 1921.

In addition to working on extracts made from the pancreas of dogs which had been made diabetic by removal of the pancreas, Collip also tested the potency of the extract in rabbits which took less time than using it on dogs. Banting's and Best's extract, the first to be used on a human subject called Leonard Thompson, produced no benefit and caused concern with the formation of of an abscess where the extract had been injected.

Eight days later, Collip developed an extract which he said was "free from all the muck."

On Monday, the 22nd of January 1922 that extract clearly demonstrated the use of insulin as a treatment for human diabetes.

Collip was also the first scientist to show that too high a dose of insulin caused the blood sugar to fall to dangerously low levels, hypoglycaemia. This is commonly called "hypo"or "insulin shock" or "insulin reaction". It is a common problem faced by patients who use insulin.

Another of Collip's experiments showed that insulin cleared the patients' urine and blood of ketones which if allowed to accumulate can be harmful.

Of his success in isolating insulin he said, "I have never had such an absolutely satisfactory experience before, namely going in a logical way from point to point in an unexplored field building absolutely solid structure all the way."

Collip together with Banting and Best were the three men to whom in 1922, the Canadian US and British patent offices granted a patent for insulin which the three immediately assigned to the University of Toronto Board of Governors, thus ensuring that no commercial interests could patent insulin for financial gain. The Board of the university was to oversee the granting of licenses to manufacturers with 50% of the profits going to the University for its research and the remainder to Banting, Best and Collip for their scientific work.

Collip had always been uncomfortable with the conflict over the insulin discovery. In later years he and Banting became friends. On what turned out to be the final evening of his life, Banting had gone to visit Collip. It was bitterly cold and Collip noticed that Banting, being his usual disorganised self, did not have any gloves. The younger man gave his sheepskin gloves to Banting. This was the ill-fated journey which ended in the tragedy of Banting's death in the plane crash in Newfoundland.

He was the only one of the four men involved in the discovery of insulin who maintained his dignity when responding to questions of priority for the success of the experiments. His usual answer was that he was "happy to let the insulin story stand on the publications by the group who collaborated in 1921–1922."

Collip devoted his entire life to medical research, mostly at McGill University. He isolated several hormones including "Premarin", one of the highest selling pharmaceutical products in the world.

He received many honours and awards and by the end of his career was recognised as a leader in the development of medical research in Canada. A book on his life and his influence on research in Canada was written by Allison Li after his death.

Collip died of a stroke in 1965. He was 72 years old.

Charles Herbert Best the Greatest Beneficiary of the Nobel Award Never to Win the Nobel Prize

When the Nobel Prize was announced Best was in Boston having been invited to speak at Harvard University. He stayed with Elliott Joslin whose elegant home (which included his office) on Bay State Road had been visited frequently by Best since their initial contact at the American Physiology Society meeting at Yale the previous year. Writing back to his fiancé Margaret Mahon, Best told her of the Boston newspapers referring to him as "the most famous medical student in the world" and the President of Harvard University Charles William Eliot repeating the description when introducing him to the students who had responded with thunderous applause. It is to his credit that in spite of his age – he was barely 22 – Best appears to have handled himself with a maturity beyond his years. As if that weren't enough, after he had spoken, Joslin read to the gathering a telegram he had just received from Frederick Banting, the winner of the Nobel Prize. The telegram read,

"I assign to Best equal share discovery insulin. Hurt that Nobel trustees did not acknowledge him, will share with him. Please read this telegram at any dinner or meeting. Banting."

Elliott Joslin read the telegram again that evening when entertaining Best and some Harvard colleagues over dinner at his home.

Joslin never commented publicly, or in any of his papers in the Joslin archives, on the controversy over the Nobel Prize not being shared with Best.

At no stage from the time of the first meeting between Banting and Best had there been any doubt as to who was the senior member of the two-man team which had embarked on the search for insulin. Neither had there been any indication at any stage that Best saw himself as doing any more than fulfilling the role of a student helping the researcher as had been suggested by his professor, James Macleod. It was, after all, a summer job and not strictly binding in any way. For instance, soon after starting, Best had gone for a 10–day military training camp. Therefore It would not be unreasonable to suggest that the "sharing" of the award was restricted, as it had to be, to giving him part of the money Banting received. It was a decision made entirely by Banting and reflected his awareness of and gratitude to his younger associate's help.

The award also included the Nobel medal and a citation which carried the name of the winner. Henry Best's book *Margaret and Charley* carries extensive records of Charles and Margaret Best's correspondence including Charles Best's views on the awarding of the Nobel Prize. Best's name as the second author was recorded in all the publications relating to the discovery of insulin by Banting.

However there was not a single nomination for Best to receive the Nobel Prize. At best he was referred to as a "collaborator" by many senior men in Toronto University including James Fitzgerald although at the time Fitzgerald was speaking about the various local honours being bestowed on Banting alone. Fitzgerald, who as Head of the Connaught Laboratories had been close to the investigative work being done on insulin from the beginning did not enter into the controversy over the sharing of the award with Best or for that matter, the inclusion of Macleod.

Apart from Banting's telegram, the first mention of Best receiving any part of the Nobel award was by his fiancé who said that her "Charlie" was more deserving of sharing the prize than James Macleod. From the Best family papers a letter dated 26 October, 1923 from Margaret to Charlie recorded her words:

"I doubt if Professor Macleod gets any joy from the use of the $20,000 because it doesn't belong to him. The honour, and the money too, would have been wonderful, Charlie, but it wouldn't have made me love you any more. So that's the main thing."

Mahon was more expansive in a letter to her uncle Bruce Morpeth Macleod in Lethbridge, Alberta on November 25, 1923.

"Dr Banting is a fine fellow and he and Charley discovered insulin. Dr Macleod was head of the department they worked in but he was absent in Europe when Insulin was discovered. They sent hopeful reports to him in Scotland but he sent back word for them not to be over-confident. Dr Macleod is an extremely clever man who had a big reputation. Ever since the experiment proved successful he has shoved himself to the front. He spent this summer in Europe and had just returned to the university after the Nobel Prize was awarded. If the Nobel Prize was given for the discovery of insulin he should have received no part of it. Dr Banting asked President Falconer or any other man to put their finger on one thing that Dr Macleod had done towards the Discovery of Insulin.

As for Collip – Dr Banting and Charlie think he is beneath contempt. He came here, after Insulin was discovered, to assist in the purification. He was given all the information about making insulin – and when he thought he had discovered a means of greater purification he actually made an attempt to leave for the States, to patent the whole thing. He was an awful ass and people here paid no attention to him until Dr Macleod handsomely divided his share of the Nobel Prize. In the clipping you sent me, Dr Macleod remarked that Collip was "entitled to an equal share of credit for his part in the work." The next day a little paragraph appeared: "The statement that Dr Collip was entitled to an equal share of credit for his part in the work was not quite properly phrased," said Dr Macleod. "It might be more accurate to say that he is entitled to a fair share of the credit. I would be glad to correct any misapprehension. If I used the word equal I should not have done so."

All this sounds as if I were fearfully bitter on the subject but I don't think about that side of it much. Charley has really had a great deal of credit and has made a great name for himself already. Ex–President Elliot of Harvard introduced him as "the greatest medical student in the world." Charley is working very hard, as always. He is in his fifth year in Medicine and has complete charge of the manufacture of insulin."

Macleod's comments appear to have been taken from a press release in an interview after the announcement of the Nobel prize. I could not find any information on how much of the prize money Macleod received was given to Collip.

Given the source of this information viz. the Best family archives, the most likely provider was Charles Best. It must be remembered that these were private conversations between him and his fiancé as were her letters to members of her family. It is equally clear that Charles Best shared and supported Banting's views on both Macleod and Collip. Banting's tirade directed at Macleod when the Nobel award was announced required James Fitzgerald's intervention to prevent a potentially disastrous event involving Canada's first Nobel Prize winner.

It is also reasonable to assume that Best had to be careful not to criticise James Macleod, his professor and supervisor of the course Best had just completed. As has been mentioned previously the subject for Best's Masters thesis was work on the insulin extract isolated by Banting and Best. It would be mischievous to suggest that Macleod wanted to familiarise himself with the entire Insulin story given that he had initially shown scant interest in Banting's proposal and had only later given begrudging approval when the results showed that success was imminent.

What is important is Mahon's emphasis, or rather a lack of it, on Best not getting part of the prize. The penultimate sentence of her note to him showed her as being not only pragmatic but more mature than her Charley. She had said, "…the honour and the money too would have been wonderful…. but would not have made me love you any more. And that's the main thing."

Were her comments an unintended trigger of Best's conviction of being denied what was rightfully his?

Best's own assessment and the one which best fits the account of the controversy was quoted in Henry Best's book. Before quoting that however, it is important to note that Henry Best himself observed when quoting the statement made to Dr W.R. Feasby who was writing Charles Best's biography which, unfortunately he did not finish before his death, "took great pains not to offend CHB and particularly MMB."

Charles Best said:

"I don't think I took it quite as seriously at that time. I don't know that I realised exactly what was happening, but it seemed to me that I had more faith in good work being its own reward, and that I would eventually get credit for the things that I had actually done."

This statement indicates that the thought of sharing the Nobel Prize with Banting had not even entered Best's mind at the time of the actual event.

One can only speculate that it was Banting's reaction to the award as well as the thoughts of Margaret Mahon and possibly, even the "label" of being a collaborator first suggested by Fitzgerald may have sowed the seeds which continued to grow and frustrated Best for the rest of his life.

There can be no doubt that Best was nearly always mentioned in the same breath as Banting. Furthermore, Banting's appreciation of and loyalty to his younger associate requires no further emphasis. Whether that justifies Best's later expectations of a share in the Nobel prize is what has been kept alive mostly by Best himself and to a lesser extent, by Henry Best. The interview with Ralph Luft, the secretary of the Nobel committee and subsequent correspondence with Henry Best has already been mentioned. Henry Best's final comment on the matter was that had there been wider consultation on Charles Best's contribution to the discovery of insulin, "perhaps the results would have been different."

It is perhaps unfortunate that according to documented sources including his own comments in the family archives and letters, Charles Best never overcame his sense of being unfairly deprived of the Nobel Prize. Even later in his more mature years during a visit to Sweden where he was entertained lavishly he commented in his family records of the hosts' generosity as possibly an attempt to assuage their guilt for not awarding him the Nobel Prize.

He was unable to accept the plain fact that he had not received a single nomination for the award. The history of the Nobel Prize is littered with the names of illustrious scientists of the calibre of Oscar Minkowski who in spite of being nominated – Minkowski was nominated six times – were not awarded the Nobel. They had the grace to accept the umpire's decision

Charles Best's reaction to this perceived injustice perhaps made him vulnerable to the judgement not only of his peers but also the readers and scholars of the history of scientific achievements in the years which have followed the discovery of insulin in 1921. It may also explain Michael Bliss's later disappointments in Charles Best's handling of the incident.

According to Henry Best the most balanced assessment in the question of credit for the discovery of insulin was made by Professor Geza Hetenyi following the controversy over the Nobel Prize being awarded to Banting and Macleod.

It was the last article written by Hetenyi, emeritus professor of medicine at the University of Ottawa, and previously a colleague of Best and a professor in the Department of Physiology at the University of Toronto from 1957 to 1970. He had also co-authored a book with G. A. Wrenshall and W.R. Feasby, *The Story of Insulin* published on the 40th anniversary of the discovery of insulin.

In an article, "Why Can't We Get It Right? Notes on the Discovery of Insulin," he judged that Best, Collip and Macleod should all be recognised as members of the team. After complimenting Michael Bliss for the "balance" he achieved when writing *The Discovery Of Insulin* published in 1982, Hetenyi levelled blunt criticism at the historian and said, "disregarding his own judgement that to allocate individual predetermined team members is gratuitous, Bliss not only tried to do this but did so with bias into subsequent papers. Again, it seems that the temptation to allocate individual credits to one or two favoured team members at the expense of others became too strong to be resisted."

Hetenyi went on to say "a further revision followed in 1993. The focus shifts to Best and his efforts to promote Banting's and his role in the discovery at the expense of Macleod's and Collip's. The paper is written with animus, for example, it is insinuated that Best and not Banting should have been on the plane that crashed in Newfoundland. No mention is made about Best's accomplishments during the war, such as directing the work on dried blood serum for military use and his service in the Navy as of 1940.... Even if occasionally Best went too far to promote his and always Banting's role in the discovery of insulin, this does not diminish his achievements."

Henry Best regarded this as the end of the account of Best's participation in, and contribution to, the discovery of insulin saying,

"Thus ended an extraordinary two and a half years at the University of Toronto, beginning with the pioneering work of Banting and Best in the summer of 1921, followed by the nerve–wracking, but exciting period of development, purification, and manufacture of insulin in 1922, to the rollercoaster ride of recognition, controversy, and honours in 1923.

Henry Best displayed his mastery of the narrative essay by ending this part of Charles Best's story on a lighter note.

"A charming and unusual honour was accorded Banting and Best in 1925 when the Ontario government named two townships after them in the Temiskaming District, west of Latchford in the mid–north of the province. Best never manage to visit "his" township as it was quite inaccessible except by canoe and several portages, but he always considered it a special honour."

Charles Best, the Final Years

From the time of the discovery of insulin and certainly after the awarding of the Nobel Prize, Frederick Banting was the one who was feted and invited to the various events and functions already described in recognition of his role in the discovery of insulin. However, once Banting had died, it was Best who was the recipient of the accolades and invitations. Macleod being an academic and having no role in treating patients with insulin, returned to Scotland a few years after the discovery. Collip was virtually unknown to the public in spite of having made significant contributions and had left Toronto before the publicity around its discovery. Thus Best was the only member of the original team left in Toronto.

More than once during the period when local honours were being showered on Banting, Best had, perhaps with some justification, felt left out. He complained to different people including Jerry Fitzgerald. It was Fitzgerald who had pointed out to the bureaucrats in the Toronto administration that Best was not an assistant but a "collaborator."

There can be no doubting Best's capabilities as a medical scientist and educator. Yet for obvious reasons his most enduring legacy is his role as an ambassador for diabetes. As the sole active and surviving member of the team associated with the discovery of insulin he was the one – the only one – commercial organisations, hospitals, universities, research centres, charities, and pharmaceutical companies (he never lost touch with them or they with him!) and numerous international organisations including the Red Cross reached out to him to participate in or provide patronage.

On 3rd September, 1924 Best married Margaret Mahon. They had been sweethearts from their time in high school. Best often told of his failure to beat Mahon in the annual school examinations. Their lifelong love for one another was like a Hollywood script and is beautifully portrayed in the book written by their second son Henry Macleod Best who was a historian.

In 1925 Best graduated from medical school at the top of his class. Following his graduation Best followed a suggestion made by Henry Dale to do postgraduate work in London, England. Henry Dale, (later Sir Henry Dale) was the Head of the National Institute for Medical Research in London. He told Best that it would be to the young graduate's advantage to spend some time in London for initial postgraduate training. Best stayed in London from 1926 to mid 1928. A qualification which for Best was a golden academic goal was a "DSc. from the University of London". When he told Dale about this, the Englishman said that although he himself was not associated with that institution but promised to see what he could do because he "knew someone there". In 1928 Best was awarded a Doctorate in Science from the University of London. Thus early in his medical career the young Charles Best had learned the power and advantages of "who you know over what you know". It is interesting that Best's son, Henry Best had noticed this quite early in his preparation for the book *Margaret and Charley* and commented that his father had recognised the value of "networking" before that word had come into common use.

Charles Best returned to Toronto as Head of the Department of Physiology. The position had fallen vacant when James Macleod had completed his tenure and returned to his native Scotland.

Macleod had recommended Best for the position even though he had no experience in administration. Best was 29 years old. Whether or not he also served as Dean of the medical faculty which was Macleod's other appointment is unclear.

In addition to his position in Toronto University Best also served as Research Director of Connaught Laboratories. Later he held several administrative positions within the university where he remained for the rest of his working life.

HEARING CHARLES BEST IN SYDNEY 100 YEARS AFTER THE DISCOVERY OF INSULIN

In Henry Best's book, I was intrigued by a reference to Charles Best delivering the Osler Oration to an English audience in 1957. Then aged 58, Best was at the peak of his career as Professor and Head of the Department of Physiology at Toronto University. He was highly respected and had been repeatedly offered positions of leadership in more prestigious institutions including some in England but had chosen to remain in Toronto.

I didn't think anymore about it at the time as I was busy looking into the controversies surrounding the Nobel Prize being divided between Banting and Macleod.

Later, the thought occurred to me that there may be a copy of the oration somewhere. I have mentioned the Osler Society in this work on more than one occasion. This very active group of men and women, mostly physicians, in addition to their interest in William Osler share an interest in medical history. As usual I consulted Professor Milton Roxanas, who is a member of the Osler Society. Might there be a copy of the lecture in one of the archives.

Securing a copy of this lecture turned out to be an interesting exercise. Neither Toronto University library or its archives, nor McGill University's library had a copy. Milton, being on the Board of Curators of the Osler Library at McGill University was kind enough to come to my rescue.

Since McGill University library did not have a copy it was suggested that there might be a copy in London. Again it was a member of the Osler Society there, Mr Richard Osborn the honorary librarian of the Club's archives who travelled to London to search for the elusive document.

The archive of the Osler Club of London is located in its Club Room at the Royal College of Physicians of London.

Yes, the library in London had a copy of the lecture by Best.

Problem solved?

Not quite.

There was indeed a copy of Charles Best's oration but it was a recorded version preserved on one of those big reels as was the practice in the mid 1950s.

Fortunately, Richard who is clearly up-to-date with the latest advances in technical matters, was able to find a young man who could convert the recording into "sound files."

The sound files were then e-mailed to me in Sydney and transcribed by Cheryl Fleming to produce a type-written sheaf of pages which in all likelihood, were like the ones which Charles Best had placed on the lectern for the Osler Oration more than 60 years ago.

Ah, the wonders of modern science – and a reminder of how much the world has moved on.

The Osler Oration 1957 Charles Best Relives the Discovery of Insulin Decades Later

Charles Best delivered the Osler Oration on the occasion of its 36th anniversary. The function was held in the historic Rembrandt Hotel which was first built in 1911. It boasts the timeless beauty of classic Edwardian architecture.

Apart from medical luminaries, the audience also included distinguished medical dignitaries, diplomats and politicians as can be gathered from the opening line of the address:

"Mr President, My Lord, Your Excellencies, Ladies and Gentlemen, It is a very great honour particularly for a Canadian to give this Osler Oration…"

Best made an important point in the first few minutes. He said:

"Most if not all rapid and dramatic additions to biological and medical knowledge rest on a foundation provided by a very large number of earlier workers. This was the case with insulin. One of my friends has recently collected the photographs of 300 individuals who have made their contributions in the field of diabetes and insulin. There have been approximately 45,000 scientific publications on insulin since of our first article in 1922 and those who are supposed to know tell us that approximately 20 million people the world over have received insulin."

Best then went on to present a brief history of diabetes before turning to the work of several scientists who had come close to developing an effective extract of insulin. He mentioned two in particular; the Roumanian scientist Nikolai Paulesco and an American, E.L. Scott.

His next comment took me by surprise because they were similar to my own impressions of James Macleod's possible lack of familiarity with the literature on this aspect of research on diabetes which I have described earlier.

Best said:

"Professor Macleod was the Head of the Department in Toronto, and a very well informed man in carbohydrate metabolism and a very cautious Scott. If Professor Macleod had known about these papers, I feel quite sure that the work in Toronto would never have started."

Macleod's had disagreed with the conclusions based on research which pointed to the presence of "a material which increased the utilisation of sugar" in pancreatic extracts. This was stated in a textbook on the subject written by Macleod which had been published just before the Second World War.

Best then repeated what were Banting's recollections of Macleod's disinterest in Banting's idea of seeking insulin in pancreatic extracts. This part of the oration ended with the following sentence:

"Writing after the discovery of insulin Professor Macleod's recollection of the encouragement he gave Banting was appreciably warmer than to my certain knowledge was the case."

Although he emphasised the importance of the team's role in the discovery, one would find it difficult to separate the contributions made by the two main participants namely Banting and himself. In fact I was left with the impression that Best gave his role greater emphasis than anyone else's including Frederick Banting's.

James Macleod's role in the insulin story was virtually identical to Banting's opinions as contained in the book by Michael Bliss and similar to the version in the Best family archives.

In the first half of the oration Best went into considerable detail in his criticism of Macleod. It would be recalled that at an earlier time his comment on the same subject had been extremely brief, almost certainly because he was Macleod's student and was depending on the professor's assessment to successfully complete his university course.

He also steered clear of the controversy over the awarding of the Nobel Prize for the discovery of insulin.

In the lecture Best made a point of stating that the lecture was not going to be published perhaps to imply that he could speak more freely without the fear of being challenged as may have happened had the material been published.

He made several claims the accuracy of which could be questioned if compared with the records preserved in archival material. One which may raise eyebrows was, "we had some troubles and disappointments, but we eventually prepared, without a single failure, potent extracts from intact pancreases of the dog on 75 consecutive occasions...."

I could find no record of such success in any of the sources including the material available online from the records of the University of Toronto archives. Several of the dogs had died during the experiments.

Nor did he mention the difficulties he got into as soon as he was put in charge of large-scale production of insulin at the Connaught Laboratories in early 1922. He did not acknowledge the help of Lilly's chemist, George Walden whose method was critical in the development of the large-scale production of the extract and which was passed on to him by the Lilly team.

In reading the transcript of the oration I was left with the impression that Best, although generous when it came to Banting could not help positioning himself as an equal contributor to the discovery of insulin.

The essential difference in the oration between his role and that of all the others especially Collip's is Best's claim of his own contribution being greater than the biochemist's and equal to Banting's. As for Macleod, Best's comments supported Banting's view that the Professor did not deserve any share of the Nobel Prize.

His criticisms of Macleod also raise questions of a different nature. According to archival material one of the last contributions Macleod made to the University of Toronto after he had returned to his native Scotland was to nominate a successor for admission to the prestigious Royal Society with the academic degree/title of FRS.

That successor was Charles Best.

The Highlights of Best's Career – in his own words.

Clearly insulin was the highpoint of Best's career as it was in the careers of all the participants in its discovery.

In February 1978, a few weeks before his death, Best spoke to his son Henry Best of his accomplishments and the highlights of his career.

Without hesitation he named insulin as the highpoint of his career. Given his association with the discovery as the main reason for the majority of his contacts for the rest of his life, one could argue that insulin was the highpoint not only of his career but indeed his whole life. Remembering that the discovery was made before he married, insulin dominated the life of not only Charles Best but also his wife's.

Although the discovery of insulin is given a mere 50 pages in Henry Best's book, reading the entire work I found very few pages where insulin or some person or matter related to it was not mentioned.

Henry Best listed the other highlights at the end of his book. These suggest that Best was drawn to his English roots. His ancestors had come from Hampshire, England.

After insulin, Best's list of the high points, in order, were the award of the Companion of Honour by her Majesty Queen Elizabeth II whom he met in a private audience, reading the lesson in St. Paul's Cathedral in the Thanksgiving Service attended by 1200 men and women who had diabetes, giving lectures at the Royal Society and to the British Diabetic Association. Best also valued his association with Henry Dale because of the seminal role played by the Englishman during the formative years of his postgraduate training (including helping him to get the D.Sc).

He did not mention the Nobel Prize.

At the back of Henry Best's book, in addition to his four earned degrees (B.A, M.A, M.B. all from the University of Toronto and D.Sc.,University of London) are Charles Best's honorary degrees, scientific medals and awards, fellowship or membership of various scientific societies in Canada, Great Britain, United States, South America, Europe, International scientific bodies, as well as academic and scientific appointments and honours.

The list occupies eight pages.

Whether Charles Best's pursuit of some of the honours, prizes, visiting professorships, academic degrees, civic honours, audiences with prominent men and women, kings and queens possibly dominated his life and, paradoxically, at least in the minds of some, may have diminished their respect for him, is for the reader to decide.

Charles Best, at least partly by an accident of history, received honours and accolades for his role in the insulin story to the end of his life.

He died at the age of 79 on 31 March, 1978, a few days after the death of his elder son Charles "Sandy" Alexander Best, who had died at the age of 46 years.

As recorded in the life history of another distinguished Canadian, William Osler, Charles Best's death was attributed to his heartbreak at his son's premature death. The actual cause as revealed at post-mortem was a ruptured aorta.

Best is invariably mentioned in the discovery of insulin with – but always after – Banting.

Fate lavished on him the spoils of victory.

Destiny denied him the glory.

THE LATER LIVES OF THE WRITERS
Henry Bruce Macleod Best (1937–2006)

Henry Best, the younger son of Charles and Margaret Best was a respected historian and academic. In addition to serving as President of the Laurentian University, he had been in the public service working as the executive assistant to the Secretary of State for External Affairs.

The 500 odd pages of Henry Best's story of his parents are dominated as much by insulin as by his parents especially his father Charles Herbert Best.

The last word on this book however, must be about Charles Best's second son Henry Bruce Macleod Best who deserves unstinting praise and admiration for his measured and largely impartial treatment of the material at his disposal. Quite apart from the challenge of deciding how much and what to leave out of the enormous volume of material, he demonstrated remarkable restraint in keeping in check his own emotions towards his parents as well as from other members of the family including his older brother Sandy. Commenting on the amount of material available, Henry Best spoke of the possibility of another member of his family writing another book about the remarkable characters one has met in *Margaret and Charlie*. And one which will doubtless include the interesting stories of Margaret and Charlie's sons, Henry and Sandy.

It is a measure of the man that Henry Best kept himself out of the story of his parents' lives. Yet he was a respected historian and academic in his own right. From 1977 to 1984, as President of Laurentian University, he had lectured in both English and French, on the history of Québec and Canadian art. Doubtless his father, who had always enjoyed the trappings of public recognition would have been proud to see Henry awarded Knight of the Order of Merit of the Republic of Italy for services to the Italian Canadian community.

Henry Best has written a beautiful story. It is a tribute to his father as well as his mother. I'm sure he has written papers, documents, reports and, perhaps books as well. But I doubt if he has written anything quite as moving as *Margaret and Charlie. The personal story of Dr Charles Best, the Co-Discoverer of Insulin.*

No one could begrudge him a moment of reflection, even wistfulness, at the end of the task he had undertaken and completed so faithfully when he looked back on his own relationship with his parents and wrote (in the third person),

"The 10 years after his father died were the best that Henry had ever experienced with his mother. She and Linda (Margaret's widowed sister) were always pleased to see him. They had long talks about all sorts of subjects.

After 1985 Henry gradually took over matters concerning the house and finances, and Margaret and Linda we are both very appreciative...

Henry asked Barbara Hazlett, from the Diabetic Clinic at the Toronto General Hospital, who had known Margaret, and Linda since she was a child, to keep an eye on them. This she faithfully, and it was she who called Henry on 26 January 1988 to say that Margaret had passed away. She died as she had hoped she would, in her own bed at home.

Thus ends the account of the remarkable times of Margaret and Charlie Best. Their story lives on in the Best Family Papers...

Little is known about Henry Best himself. Sadly, on Good Friday, April 9, 2004 less than a year after the publication of the book, Henry Best died aged 69. His obituary listed his many scholastic accomplishments including a doctorate in history and his capacity for administration. Doubtless his father, who had enjoyed the trappings of public recognition, would have been proud to see Henry awarded Knight of the Order of Merit of the Republic of Italy for services to the Italian Canadian community.

Henry Best's tender reflections on his parents are among the most moving passages in the book. It was he who had cared for them in the final years of their lives.

Three years after completing this book Henry Best died at the age of 69 years.

My own impressions on reading the book, and referring to it many times during this work, were of Henry perhaps being the quiet achiever while his brother Sandy, also accomplished in his own field including politics, was more "visible" of the two, at least in the public eye.

I was reminded of an apocryphal tale recounted by a prophet 2000 years ago which spoke of an adventurous son whose brother's quiet and loyal and enduring devotion towards his parents may perhaps have been taken for granted.

John William Michael Bliss (1941–2017)

Michael Bliss, like Henry Best was a historian. His father and brother were doctors. His earlier works were on topics of Canadian business and politics.

In 1982 at the age of 41 Bliss wrote *The Discovery of Insulin.* It was his first "medical" book. Fascinated by the enigmatic Frederick Banting, Bliss wrote a book on the discoverer of insulin two years later.

In 1996 Bliss had joined the Osler Society. Although he does not mention his membership directly, he does acknowledge the assistance of the Osler libraries in McGill University as well as in London England in his research for his next book.

In 1999, he wrote *William Osler: A Life in Medicine.* Perhaps more readable than the Pulitzer prize winning two – volume work on Osler by Harvey Cushing written 70 years earlier, Bliss's work revived an interest in the much admired physician.

His studies on Osler had introduced him to the brilliant and unpredictable pioneer neurosurgeon, Harvey Cushing, the subject of his last medical biography.

Harvey Cushing : A Life in Surgery written in 2005 is, in my opinion, his finest work.

Six out of the twelve books he wrote were on medical subjects, mostly biographies. It is said that in his later years Biss wanted to be thought of as a "medical biographer."

The work on Osler had brought him into contact with the Osler Society, a group mostly made up of physicians interested in medical history in general and Osler in particular. Bliss was popular with, and respected by this group. In *Sir William Osler An Encyclopaedia,* edited by Charles S. Bryan which was published by Norman Publishing in 2020, Bliss is included in the list of distinguished men to whom this impressive work is dedicated.

The Early Challenges for Patients Using Insulin

The euphoria caused by the announcement of the discovery overshadowed some of the practical problems associated with the use of insulin.

Learning to use insulin when it first became available in the 1920s – first in Toronto, then in the neighbouring parts of Canada, before reaching the shores of the United States in 1924 and in England and Europe at around the same time, presented many challenges for the patient and his carers. The children needed their parents' help in getting the daily injections. Those fortunate – or wealthy – enough to acquire the services of teaching nurses were few in number. So, for that matter, were teaching nurses.

Opportunities to learn the practical aspects of treating diabetes now included a raft of new information and practices including a method for testing urine samples for sugar, the care and use of insulin syringes and needles, and storing insulin, to name just some of the requirements.

In the early years, in addition to the treating physician learning the basics of caring for a patient with insulin, the patient himself and, in the case of children, one or both parents had to become proficient in the day - to - day care of the diabetic child.

Elliott Joslin, the Boston physician who had pioneered many aspects of diabetes care including the training of teaching nurses, had written a manual for the instruction of patients and doctors because both needed guidance especially when insulin was introduced.

He emphasised the importance of understanding the basics for which his instruction manuals became popular with the patients as well as their carers.

The correct dose of insulin had to be determined for each diabetic. This required learning the method of testing for the presence of sugar (glucose) in the urine and in later years, its level in the blood. Thus, starting treatment in a diabetic was a challenge for the patient and, in many cases, also for the doctor.

The importance of education for the patient and the physician in the treatment of diabetes is as important today is it was in 1922. With increasing understanding of the diabetic condition, even if incomplete, continuing education of those suffering from the condition is even more important.

It must also be remembered that doctors were also entirely inexperienced in the use of insulin at that time. The need for educational programs for patients as well as medical staff including physicians, nurses and dieticians was recognised early. The family records of Charles Best make mention of his father, a general practitioner, coming to Toronto to learn how to treat diabetes very soon after the discovery of insulin.

Many diabetics, adults and children were, and still are, fearful of daily injections usually three or four times every 24 hours.

In the early years some patients including children had to have injections during the night.

The effect of the extract of insulin in the early years often did not last much more than one or two hours.

Infections at the site of injections troubled many especially those in whom they progressed to large abscesses. Other local problems at the site of injections were allergic reactions to the insulin preparation.

Low blood sugar reactions, hypoglycaemia also frequently referred to as "hypos" are still a challenge in the day-to-day management of diabetes.

The less educated, especially in under-developed countries simply could not cope with the amount of information and knowledge needed for treating their diabetes. Of course the less educated can be found in many countries, not just in the Third world. During my time in Boston I frequently came across patients from the poorer suburbs who simply did not have the educational background to grasp the basic information on diabetes.

Improvements in the manufacture of needles and syringes as well as methods of measuring glucose levels in the blood made the management of diabetes much simpler than it was in the early days. Now, automated insulin delivery systems spare the diabetic the pain and inconvenience of insulin injections. This is a far cry from the many challenges faced by the diabetic of the 1920s.

Poverty compounds the difficulties. In some instances even the distances diabetics had to travel to the nearest medical facilities were beyond their means. This was an important issue especially in the less developed countries. In some of these countries I came across instances of diabetic children being abandoned by their parents to the care of the hospital because it was impossible for them to travel the distances involved and also to pay for treatment including the purchase of insulin.

Insulin – the tip of an iceberg

In the minds of scholars of medical history the discovery of insulin by the team in Toronto may complete the chapter on the pursuit of the "elusive internal secretion." The dramatic benefits of the reduction in blood sugar made possible by insulin cannot be overstated but the euphoria caused by the announcement of the discovery drowned out the practical problems associated with the use of insulin. Very early in the course of using insulin several practical problems associated with its use quickly brought the realisation that the dramatic results came at a cost.

It did not take long for the patients and doctors to see that hand-in-hand with the benefits of insulin came several challenges and that insulin was in fact the tip of an iceberg.

For the practising physician it was just the beginning of the quest for the treatment of diabetes.

So, how good was the Nobel Prize-winning insulin extract when it came to its practical, every day use as a treatment for diabetes?

The short answer is "not very good."

Insulin has been called *"a daily miracle."*

Yes, it is that, but the miracle came with challenges some of which are described here.

The introduction of insulin in the treatment of diabetes posed several challenges which confronted a diabetic every day, in fact, several times every day. The various aspects of treatment included planning and supervising the diet, measuring and recording the level of sugar in the urine and blood as well as planning the daily activities of the patient required attention and often supervision, several times every day.

The effects of the early preparations of insulin lasted no more than 3 to 4 hours, sometimes even less. Therefore the patient was subjected to several injections each day and sometimes even during the night.

A particularly troubling problem of using insulin which remains unsolved has been the necessity for giving it into the skin and muscle of the patient by subcutaneous (under the skin) injection. This has remained the practice and has been satisfactory from the point of view of the effect of insulin which is absorbed quickly into the bloodstream through the numerous finer branches of the bigger arteries situated in the deeper layers of muscles in the upper and lower limbs. Unfortunately however, injections have always been a challenge as much from the very thought of giving or receiving an injection as from the actual procedure.

Improvements through advances in technology have made injections much less troublesome with the finer and better designed needles causing less pain. Still, not only the patient but, in the case of children, to the parents also the very thought of injecting the children was and in many instances remains even today, a daily heartache.

Further challenges arose from the unpredictability of the effectiveness of different batches of insulin. For example the product from the laboratory of the Lilly Company often differed from that produced in Toronto's Connaught Laboratories.

It soon became clear that the practical application of the insulin extract discovered by Banting and his colleagues was neither a panacea nor a miracle cure.

That the different chemical steps in refining –"purifying"– the extract were of critical importance had been realised mainly by Bertram Collip in the original team of researchers. He had used a different concentration of alcohol when preparing the extract which, unlike the batches produced by Charles Best, was the first to demonstrate a beneficial effect on a patient with diabetes.

This was the extract which at 11 o'clock in the morning of Monday, January 22nd, 1922 was injected in the arm of Leonard Thompson, the first human diabetic on whom insulin produced effects to the satisfaction of the physicians who were treating Thompson in hospital.

The extract made by Best, and much trumpeted by the Toronto Star, had been injected into the same patient a few weeks earlier. It had failed dismally.

As related earlier, the group witnessing the successful injection did not include Banting because he had been banned by Duncan Graham from attending, let alone giving the injection, as had been Banting's dream.

Banting never forgot nor forgave being barred from participating in that historic "clinical trial." It had been part of his ambition, his dream.

The Wider Distribution of Insulin

"The biggest thing that ever happened in medicine."
Josiah Lilly, August 1923.

Looking at the various laboratories, drug houses and research facilities especially in North America and England it is clear that the main supplier of insulin of reliable quality was the Lilly Company. From the very beginning Clowse and the two Lillys, Josiah and Eli, had a clear vision of the size of the market for the product in the United States alone.

Their unerring foresight came to dramatic fruition in the second half of 1923.

According to Bliss, within 12 to 18 months of the beginning of the process to commercialise the manufacture of insulin, around 7000 American physicians were prescribing the hormone for their patients. By September 1923 some 20,000 Americans were receiving several injections of insulin each day.

Clowse, with his knack for nurturing, then maintaining a close relationship with physicians who had large numbers of diabetics in their care such as Joslin and Allen had personally assured them of a reliable supply of insulin from Lilly as early as July 1922.

That the Lilly operatives were only just beginning to fully grasp the potential of their new product in July/August 1923 is expressed in a letter from the owner Josiah K. Lilly to Clowse at that time.

He said, "I am almost overwhelmed with this tremendous situation and experience some difficulty in keeping my feet on the ground and my brain in normal operation.... MacDonald (a doctor in Indianapolis) says it looks to him that it's the biggest thing that ever happened in medicine, and that is saying a good deal because some very big things have happened in medicine. You have certainly entered the holy of holies, and are sitting on the throne with the elect. It is a marvellous development and I rejoice in it."

Even though the University of Toronto generously granted patents to many individuals and companies throughout Canada and the United States, it was the Lilly company which remained the major supplier of insulin to the drug houses of the United States, Canada as well as, much to the chagrin of the British drug houses, to the pharmacies in Britain.

The euphoria following the discovery of insulin had blinded many of the main players including the discoverers to the very practical considerations of getting the product to where it was needed most namely the patient. As has been mentioned more than once, only Banting from the group involved in the discovery was single-minded in his determination to getting the extract to patients with diabetes. He was not particularly interested in the commercial side of the exercise.

However the commercial potential of insulin had not escaped the notice of a canny Englishman called J. A. Clowse, the Research Director of Lilly.

Clowse, an experienced researcher in his own right had recognised, perhaps earlier than anyone, the potential commercial benefits of providing insulin to the thousands of diabetics not only in the United States but all around the world.

As in many human pursuits including commercial enterprise, "timing is everything".

Clowse moved quickly.

One of the brightest chemists in the research division of Lily was a young man called George Walden. Clowse freed him from all his other duties and instructed him to devote all his time to developing a reliable method of producing insulin of a consistent strength so that it's effect on the blood sugar of diabetics would be reliable and predictable.

Walden recognised the urgency of the project. However he was a methodical and disciplined researcher. Working long hours Walden studied every step of extract production. Working at a feverish pace between October and December 1922, he produced the first reliable supply of insulin. Furthermore, the insulin produced by Lilly was more stable, and ten to a hundred times purer than any other preparation at that time.

The spectacular success of the Lilly insulin was beyond all of Clowse's expectations. So elated was he that in March 1923 Clowse in a letter to Henry Dale boasted of their huge reserves of insulin.

"We can produce in Indianapolis a sufficient amount of "Iletin" (Lilly's brand name for insulin) to supply the entire needs of the civilised world."

There was little love lost between the two Englishmen. Dale held himself as being superior to Clowse because of the latter's association with "business." Never mind that Dale had earlier worked for the well-known British pharmaceutical firm Burroughs Wellcome for a period. He was now part of the research group in London and later headed the National Institute for Medical Research. He had devoted most of his life to research and was rewarded with the Nobel Prize in 1936. However when it came to business and commercial acumen Dale was no match for Clowse.

Dale was not to know that the patent for producing insulin established as an "indenture"between the Board of Governors of the University of Toronto and Eli Lilly and Company was to expire at the end of 12 months on 30 May 1923.

The feverish pursuit of commercial advantage and the dog - eat - dog mentality especially between the Lilly and the British team obscured the very real issue of inconsistent effects of the various insulin preparations in the laboratories of the other parties involved.

Another of the troublesome problems with the use of insulin in the early days and one which remains a challenge, was the effect of blood glucose levels dropping below normal levels producing what is usually referred to as "hypos". These cause symptoms which may range from mild problems like slight dizziness to medical emergencies including loss of consciousness. In the early days, a patient treated by Dr Robert Williams in Rochester was "so lifeless that the chief of our surgical staff pronounced him dead.

We immediately restored him by the injection of some glucose, and it was looked upon as a miracle in the hospital."

It was a difficult period for the diabetic whose hopes had been raised by the discovery of insulin in 1922. It was also a frustrating time for physicians treating diabetes. It became clear that insulin in the form available at that time provided only part of the solution and more work remained to be done. Two early challenges were firstly, to refine the actual process of producing the extract and secondly, to develop a preparation of insulin which would last longer than 2 to 3 hours.

It also became clear that unless the insulin preparations available to the patient could produce consistent and predictable results regardless of where they were manufactured, there would be difficulties in the treatment of individual patients. Furthermore, unless all the preparations marketed by the different companies produced predictable degrees of reduction in the blood sugar the difficulties for diabetics and the doctors treating them would persist. Clearly the methods of extraction, purification and concentration of the hormone had to be, not only improved but, standardised.

Standardisation of Insulin

Initially it was thought that the reasons for the inconsistency were due to differences in the methods of extracting insulin produced by the Lilly and Connaught Laboratories. Then Lilly found that there were differences between batches produced in a laboratory. Frustratingly, sometimes the differences amounted to a 20% variation in the effectiveness of insulin as measured by the reduction in the blood sugar. Clearly this was a problem which had to be solved if insulin was going to be suitable for regular daily use in the treatment of diabetes.

The foresight of Clowse in appointing Walden had paid off handsomely. The critical finding made by Walden was that the degree of acidity (technically referred to as the pH) differed from batch to batch. This had produced the unpredictable effects of the insulin extracts made in Connaught Laboratories as well in Dale's Laboratories in London, England. Once the acidity was controlled by using the method perfected in the Lilly laboratories, the effect of insulin became consistent and therefore predictable. Furthermore, to Walden's delight, Insulin made with this method produced a more potent product than any previous batches.

What has been mentioned previously was the generosity of the different groups working on insulin as far as sharing their information with other workers in the same field.

(As you will read later, this was a far cry from the fierce competition between the different groups involved in the discovery of modern insulin. It was enough to land one of them in the Emergency Unit of a local hospital.)

As had been done by the Toronto researchers with the Danish team headed by August Krogh, Lilly through Clowse, provided the information on the extraction method discovered by Walden to the English team in London.

In summary then, many of the early problems as described above had been addressed with varying degrees of success – with one exception. This was the effect of insulin lasting at best only 3 to 4 hours, often only two hours. The practical result of this was the necessity for injections two, three or even four times every day. Sometimes the injections had to be given during the night. Quite apart from the pain was the necessity for assistance from whoever was tasked with helping the patient especially children with managing their diabetes..

It was generally agreed that finding a way to make the effect of injected insulin last longer was perhaps the most important improvement to be pursued by the scientists involved in research on insulin.

It is important to remember that for 15 years after the discovery of insulin patients had to be injected up to 4 times each day. A new discovery was to change that.

THE SECOND GREAT DISCOVERY IN THE INSULIN STORY

".... the action of insulin, although wonderful, lasted only a few hours and was also unlike nature in that it caused sudden and often serious falls of the sugar in the blood..."
    A Diabetic Manual for the Mutual Use of Doctor and Patient. (Sixth edition). 1937. Elliott P. Joslin.

A Trout Fisherman in the Insulin Story

"To be a *shikari* (hunter) was a very great thing in Kashmir ....and to be a good *shikari* was a dedication, beyond imitating or mistaking."
    Robin Levett, *The Shikari* 1997.

Fishing for trout is one of the most popular sports and hobbies throughout the world. The intelligence, cunning and wiles of the trout are well known to those familiar with it. For some, it is a lifelong pursuit, their interest verging on religious fervour. The habits of one particular trout are beautifully described in the book *The Shikari* by Robin Levett. It is an account of the pursuit of one very cunning fish in a mountain stream in Kashmir with the guidance of a shikari who had devoted his entire life to learning the habits of the fish and which he used in his occupation as a professional guide for tourists wanting to experience the joys of the sport.

An early challenge for patients who needed insulin was that its effect didn't last longer than about three hours, often even less. The patient had to be injected two or three, even four times every day. An early attempt to overcome this was to inject larger quantities of insulin which unfortunately resulted in much of the insulin being lost in the urine or at other times lowering the blood sugar to levels which caused dizziness, even unconsciousness.

The solution to this problem brings to the stage an earlier individual in the *dramatis personae* of the insulin story.

Hans Christian Hagedorn, the chemist who, with August Krogh, had earlier established the first pharmaceutical company to produce insulin in Denmark, was also a trout fisherman.

Hagedorn had never forgotten the joy of watching trout in the streams and rivers of his native land during his childhood. He had frequented the streams and rivers where the cool waterways provided an attractive habitat for the river trout. Fish had been used in experimental studies on carbohydrate metabolism including insulin for many workers. Macleod of the Toronto group had conducted studies on carbohydrate metabolism including attempts at isolating insulin in fish even after the discovery of insulin from beef pancreas by Banting and Best. Charles Best in his family archives had dismissed Macleod's belief in the practical use of fish insulin as being "too expensive."

Hagedorn was aware of the problems caused by the frequent injections of insulin. In early 1930s he became interested in modifying the absorption of insulin from the subcutaneous tissue where it was deposited by injection. Earlier research had shown that when insulin preparations were contaminated by proteins, in addition to causing local irritation, the absorption of insulin was slowed. He decided that his first project was to find a protein which did not cause local irritation when injected into the skin.

Protamine was a protein which was found in the sperm of fish and had been described by the Swiss physician Johannes Friederich

Miescher (1844–1895) in 1868. Hagedorn discovered that protamine was what he needed. The trout fisherman was delighted to discover that protamine was especially plentiful in the sperm of the trout. Hagedorn used the sperm of the rainbow trout, *salmo iridius,* a species which was plentiful throughout Scandinavia.

Adding protamine to insulin changed the nature of insulin which turned into small microscopic clumps. Clumps of insulin in the bloodstream took longer to dissolve and so the effect of insulin could be prolonged. When injected under the skin, as it was in patients with diabetes, it was absorbed even more slowly than the quick-acting (soluble) insulin which was at that time in general use.

In 1936 Hagedorn introduced to the treatment of diabetes a new insulin compound namely Protamine insulin. It had been used in Denmark since 1934, marketed as Leo "insulin retard".

A further discovery revealing that insulin was markedly improved with the addition of a small amount of zinc was based on the work of D.A. Scott of Toronto. Scott, as early as 1935, had shown that crystalline insulin was in fact a chemical compound of zinc and insulin namely, zinc insulinate. He had discovered that the addition of traces of zinc produced zinc protamine insulin in suspension which was more stable and had a more prolonged effect than any previous preparation including the Protamine insulin marketed by Hagedorn. Further trials established the fact that protamine zinc insulin, as the new preparation was called, was more stable and more prolonged in its action than any previously discovered preparation including the one being marketed by Hagedorn.

Another advantage of the new preparation was that it was stable in suspension in a bottle which simply had to be shaken for the liquid to be thoroughly mixed before being drawn up and injected. The previous preparation of protein insulin without the addition of zinc had required the insulin to be issued in two bottles, one containing the insulin and the other a buffer (a liquid which when added to the Insulin made it stable). The insulin and the buffer had to be drawn up separately and mixed in the syringe before injection.

The introduction of Protamine Zinc Insulin in 1936 was revolutionary from the point of view of the diabetic. For the first time since their introduction in 1922–23 insulin injections did not have to be given every 2 to 3 hours, sometimes even as frequently as every hour to keep the blood sugar within manageable levels. Instead the new preparation had to be given just once a day.

Elliott Joslin, who was caring for perhaps the largest number of insulin-treated diabetics in that part of the world, hailed Hagedorn's contribution as a new era in the evolution of diabetes care. In the sixth edition of *The Treatment of Diabetes Mellitus* published in 1937, the year after the introduction of PZI he wrote:

"Protamine insulin constitutes the most notable advance in the treatment of diabetes since the discovery of insulin in 1921. The action of regular insulin was dramatic in lowering the blood sugar and promoting the utilisation of carbohydrates with all that implies, but the effect was temporary and for adequate control of most cases of diabetes two, three, and even four injections needed to be given daily. Protamine Zinc Insulin changed that with the number of injections reduced to once a day."

Naturally the use of protamine zinc insulin was a radical improvement in the treatment of diabetes by making it possible, for the very first time, to reduce the number of injections needing to be given to a diabetic. It was widely adopted In the treatment of insulin– requiring diabetics throughout the world.

(I found an interesting comment on the introduction of Protamine Zinc Insulin by Robert Lawrence, whose story has been described in this account at the time of the discovery of insulin. Lawrence commented on the use of the term "ordinary insulin" which was a term used for short-acting insulin preparations before the addition of Protamine. To emphasise that he himself having been rescued by Insulin, had not forgotten the wonder of the discovery brought forth his comment, "Of course there is no such thing as *ordinary* insulin. Insulin is *extraordinary*.")

Improvements in insulin preparations

The introduction of Protamine Zinc Insulin (PZI) in 1936 meant that the diabetic had two preparations of insulin, the short acting "soluble" or "regular" insulin which usually lasted for 3 to 4 hours and PZI which usually lasted for more than 24 hours. The need for further work in this area was highlighted by the early discovery that in some patients Protamine Zinc Insulin kept the blood sugar down for longer than 24 hours, occasionally up to 36 hours. Therefore if such a patient received a second dose of insulin the following day the combined effects of the two injections often led to profound lowering of blood sugar which caused dizziness and, in some cases, loss of consciousness. In the occasional patient such a reaction resulted in a fit like that seen in people suffering from epilepsy. This gave rise to the false belief that diabetics were prone to epilepsy.

In the early years when soluble insulin was the only preparation available –14 years, and then between the introduction of PZI and the medium-acting preparations, another 14 years, it isn't difficult to realise the challenges faced by the patient and his carers before the more suitable and convenient preparations became available. The challenge of daily injections and the associated problems such as the pain sustained especially by children needing several injections each day was to remain a problem for the patient and, especially in the young, their parents and health professionals for years to come.

Although Hagedorn is credited with the introduction of this new preparation, Protamine Zinc Insulin, significant contributions to the eventual preparation for clinical use owed its development to other workers particularly D.A. Scott working at the Connaught Laboratories where Banting and Best had worked on the original insulin extract. Scott and Fisher had found that by adding an infinitely small amount of zinc to insulin they could produce a suspension of protein/insulin crystals which dissolved slowly, delaying the breakdown of the combination of insulin and protamine and slowing the absorption of insulin into the circulation.

From 1921 when the first preparations of insulin were developed in Toronto to 1936 when Hagedorn produced PZI the diabetic was totally reliant on these two preparations. However the trout fisherman's contribution initiated a concerted effort on the part of chemists and pharmaceutical companies to develop more preparations of insulin.

Clearly intermediate acting preparations of insulin were needed.

The Development of Medium–Duration Insulin Preparations

Hagedorn had continued to work on insulin and in 1946 developed neutral Protamine insulin which he called NPH, (Neutral Protamine Hagedorn) also called Isophane insulin because of the "isophane" combination of protamine and insulin without any surplus of either.

Another practical advantage of Isophane insulin was that unlike PZI, Isophane insulin could be mixed with the quick-acting "soluble" insulin in the same syringe so the patient could have both preparations in a single injection and not two injections as was necessary with PZI.

The development of medium–duration insulins like isophane used in combination with short–acting preparations like soluble insulin lead to widespread use of these by diabetic patients around the world and remains the practice in many countries to this day.

By 1950 the range of Insulins used was largely a combination of the short and medium acting preparations. PZI was largely replaced by these.

This table summarises the history of the newer preparations. It is taken from the Diabetic Manual by E.P. Joslin 1959.

Type of insulin	Yr. marketed	Maximum effect	Duration of effect
Regular	1922	1–2	6
Crystalline	1936	1–2	7
Protamine zinc	1936	12	26–48
Globin	1939	8–10	18–24
NPH	1950	8–10	26–30
Lente	1954	8–10	26–30
Semi Lente	1954	Slow	12–18
Ultra Lente	1954	Very slow	36

NPH insulin originally from animal sources has arguably been the most successful preparation for the treatment of Type-One diabetes. It is still used although no longer sourced from animals alone. This will be discussed later in the insulin story. It must be emphasised however that insulin sourced from animals is still used in many countries largely because some of the newer insulin preparations are expensive.

From the patients' point of view there is general agreement that the first major improvement was the development of longer acting preparations which reduced the need for several injections every day. One can also appreciate the joy of doctors engaged in treating diabetics and praising the efforts of men like Hagedorn.

This brief description of the development of insulin produced in Toronto in the 1920s when seen in the light of the progress made over the many decades since highlights the remarkable advances made in this area through the work of scientists especially in the discipline of chemistry. Hagedorn remained involved in the treatment of diabetes in general and the use of insulin in particular to the end of his life. The unerring insight of Marie Krogh in her decision to harness the talents and capabilities of Hans Christian Hagedorn will form part of an essay on some of the remarkable women who feature in the insulin story later in this account.

Thus, in 1936, the treatment of diabetes with insulin consisted of two preparations namely "regular" or soluble insulin which lasted 3 to 4 hours and, at the other end of the spectrum, PZ I which lasted for more than 24 hours.

Emphasising the need for further work in this area was highlighted when it was discovered that in some patients PZI lasted even longer than 24 hours – up to 36 hours. If a patient on PZI insulin had a second dose of insulin on the day after the first injection, the accumulated effects of the two doses resulted in serious reductions in the blood glucose levels causing profound hypoglycaemic reactions. This, in some patients, caused seizures as seen in epilepsy giving rise to the false belief that diabetics were prone to epilepsy.

Clearly intermediate acting preparations of insulin were needed. Fortunately research in further modifications of insulin and protamine and other agents continued to be explored in the late 1930s and 1940s. This led to the development of intermediate acting preparations such as Globin insulin (which used protein and zinc) and Lente Insulin (which used zinc and acetate in a solution which was of the same acidity as blood). Short–acting semilente, and the long-acting Ultra Lente completed the full range of Lente insulins.

In the 1950s, Hagedorn developed Neutral Protamine Hagedorn (NPH) also called Isophane insulin (because of the "isophane" combination of both protamine and insulin without any surplus of either) which was the most popular and in many ways the first intermediate acting insulin which had a slower onset and a longer duration of action compared with the regular insulin available at that time.

Unlike, PZI, Isophane insulin could be mixed with quick-acting insulin in the same syringe so the patient could have both preparations in a single injection and not two injections as was necessary with PZI.

By 1950 the range of insulin preparations used In the day-to-day management of patients with diabetes diabetes was largely a combination of the short and medium acting preparations. PZI was largely replaced by these these.

The pioneering work of Hagedorn however, was not forgotten largely because of his continuing contributions to and life-long interest in the evolution of scientific advances in the treatment of diabetes as well as the commercial aspects of marketing insulin.

NPH insulin has arguably been the most successful formulation of insulin for use in diabetic patients and is still used today although no longer sourced from animals in all the countries.

The modern insulin preparations prepared through technological advances are currently more expensive than the earlier varieties. This has been one of the reasons for the limited use in the poorer countries.

This brief description of the development of insulin originally produced by Banting and Best in the early 1920s, when seen in the light of its development over the decades since, reveals the remarkable advances in that aspect of the treatment of the patient suffering from diabetes.

Of course insulin did not solve all the problems which continue to challenge diabetics and those involved in caring for them. Ironically, complications resulting from diabetes of long duration largely achieved through the use of insulin are now a major cause of hospitalisation and a challenge for patients, their carers as well as the providers of health care.

The discovery of insulin by Banting and his colleagues in Toronto did not mark the end of the insulin story. In fact It could be argued that the pursuit of insulin by Banting had started with the single purpose of finding a treatment for diabetes. Therefore one could regard the discovery and development of the extract including its purification as part of the original exercise. The team led by Banting assisted by Best and later by Collip was followed by the participation of other workers especially David Scott at Connaught Laboratories.

Within 12 months of the original discovery the need for large – scale production of insulin for distribution beyond Toronto and Canada became the overriding concern of the team. The dramatic effects of the pancreatic extract on the host of diabetics around the world dominated the thinking of physicians treating the condition to say nothing of the emotional outpourings of euphoric patients, their relatives and carers worldwide.

The practising physician, as I have emphasised, favours the pragmatic, even empirical treatment as long as it "works." Scientific accuracy and precision or "purity", take second-place to achieving relief for the patient.

In effect, once insulin was made available for treatment, most of the attention was devoted to its effects on patients with diabetes.

Scientific investigations into the actual chemical and molecular nature of insulin receded into the background.

However this did not mean that laboratory research stopped – only that it receded into the background of public attention.

The next story illustrates that diminishing attention, even in scientific circles, did not totally stifle the interest in trying to solve the mystery of the actual chemical and molecular nature of insulin.

PART FIVE
THE MODERN INSULIN

THE INSULIN STORY'S FORGOTTEN HERO

John Jacob Abel (1857–1938)

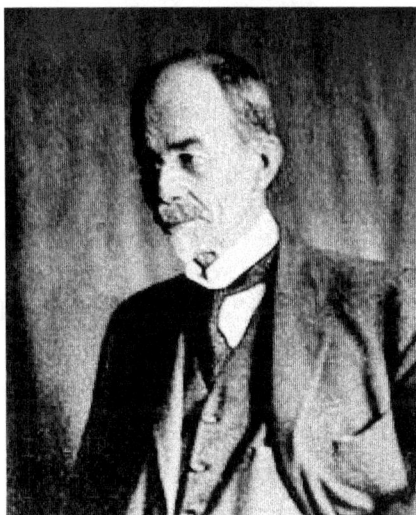

John J Abel isolated insulin crystals.

"Will attack insulin."

John J. Abel. 1921.

The prevailing scientific thought on the nature of insulin was that it was carried by a protein and insulin itself was "attached" or "stuck" to the protein surface. The scientific term for this type of association/attachment is *adsorption* and the "Adsorption Theory" held sway for many years after the dramatic events of the summers of 1921 and 1922 in Toronto.

John Jacob Abel was born in 1857 in Cleveland, Ohio. His parents were farmers of German ancestry. Abel attended the University of Michigan and at the age of 22 accepted the position of principal of a high school in Indiana. Three years later he returned to the university to study physiology and chemistry and graduated in 1883. Abel then travelled to Europe where he spent a total of nearly 7 years in central Europe spending periods with many universities with renowned medical schools and studying under the tutorship of some of the giants of medicine and physiology. He studied chemistry, pathology and clinical medicine. This period proved to be life-changing as he pursued courses in several branches of science. He studied physiology at University of Leipzig followed by an intensive two – year period in the winter of 1886 and 1887 at the University of Strasbourg. Studying internal medicine under the tutorship of Adolph Kussmaul and pathology and infectious diseases with the guidance of Friederich von Recklinghausen was a life–changing experience for Abel. The University of Strasbourg was a revered cradle of scientific thought and education. It counted amongst its alumni a formidable array of intellectual giants including Bernhard Naunyn, and Louis Pasteur who went on to become respected and influential figures in Europe's medical and scientific communities. The name of Adolph Kussmaul is familiar to all physicians because of the description of a change in the pattern of breathing which takes place when a diabetic goes into life-threatening diabetic coma.

Strasbourg was not only a nursery for medical scientists but also others such as the highly respected and multi-talented Albert Schweitzer, the Nobel laureate with a triple doctorate (theology music and medicine) who with his wife, a nurse, built and ran a hospital and devoted his life to providing medical care to natives in Lambarene, a village in a remote region of Africa.

Abel finished his time with Kussmaul after graduating with an MD. This broad scientific education and experience as well as the influence of brilliant teachers in Germany was to stand him in good stead for his wide-ranging scientific endeavours and experiments over the next 50 years.

This long period in Europe created in him a lasting relationship with many of his teachers especially in Germany. Remember his ancestral connections were in Rhineland. However nobody who knew Abel personally could doubt the influence of America, the land of his birth and upbringing. "He remained staunchly American in sentiment and habit of mind."

In 1890 Abel started as a Professor of Pharmacology at the University of Michigan where he established the Department of Pharmacology, the first of its kind in North America.

In 1893 he was invited by William Osler to join the Medical faculty at Johns Hopkins as its first full professor of pharmacology. Abel occupied this position for the next 50 years to the end of his life.

His interest in insulin started with an invitation by his friend Arthur Noyes who had received a grant from the Carnegie Corporation for research into insulin following its discovery by Banting in Toronto in 1921. After preliminary studies including experiments on insulin Abel decided to accept Noyes's invitation. His reply contained a brief and pithy statement:

"Will attack insulin, writing. JJ Abel."

The initial part of his work consisted of purifying insulin extract, an exercise which had occupied the minds and time of the original researchers in Toronto as detailed earlier in this account. Abel's attempts to verify insulin included measuring the sulphur content of his extract which revealed that the higher the sulphur content the greater the activity of the extract. This was the first clear evidence on the structure of insulin namely that sulphur is an integral part of the insulin molecule.

A remarkable event in December 1925 was akin to an epiphany for the hard-working and brilliant scientist. In December 1925

Abel was captivated by a vision which he said was "one of the most beautiful sites of my life."

What he had seen were glistening crystals of insulin on the inside surface of a test tube.

He sent a preliminary report which was published in the Proceedings of the National Academy of Sciences in February 1926 and described "a beautiful biuret reaction" a test which demonstrated that insulin was a protein. The title of the paper was "Crystalline Insulin."

This was the first time that insulin was recognised as a protein and not something that was being *carried* by a protein. The effects of insulin (on blood sugar levels) which were the reason for its newfound fame following the discovery in Toronto were still being attributed to a protein upon which Insulin was "adsorbed". This was the prevailing view on the physiological role of proteins at that time. It was an entirely new concept because scientific thought at that time maintained that proteins did not possess the specific physiological capabilities as shown by a hormone such as insulin. To call Abel's findings revolutionary would be an understatement. Therefore it was not surprising that Abel himself began to doubt the validity of his findings. Although a pharmacologist by training he was hesitant to believe that insulin possessed such unique and hitherto undescribed effects when injected into a diabetic as shown in his experiments.

Abel's work eventually came to be recognised as the first to demonstrate that insulin, a hormone was a protein which exerted specific and predictable effects.

Regardless of the reaction of his peers, many young researchers came to Abel's laboratory and studied the newly crystallised hormone under his guidance.

It is interesting that the medical fraternity was also reluctant to accept a proposition contrary to the status quo namely that insulin was a protein which possessed specific properties of its own. The Joslin textbook seemed almost hesitant to dismiss the Adsorption Theory. Even in the final edition, the 10th, published in 1959 more than 20 years after Abel had reported his findings, Joslin said,

"Crystalline insulin gives all the reactions of a typical protein."

He then went on to describe various reactions of proteins to acids and alkalis before stating that it "seemed unlikely that the active principle was merely adsorbed on the protein. Rather, it seemed fairly certain that the protein was identical with the hormone, insulin."

So Joslin, one of the most experienced specialists in diabetes, considered that insulin being a protein was only "fairly certain."

There is no mention of Abel in the book by Bliss, nor in the material contained in Henry Best's work based on Charles Best's notes and recollections.

A final incident of historical interest is an event which befell Abel a few months after he had isolated the insulin crystals.

In trying to answer the criticisms of his opponents who held to the Adsorption Theory, Abel was frustrated by an unforeseen occurrence. Between March 1926 and January 1927, for reasons he could not fathom, Abel lost the ability to crystallise insulin.

He had been working on insulin supplied by the Lilly Company which had not told Abel that the insulin they had given him was a mixture of beef and pork. Abel thought that this was the reason but many years later, a more likely cause was suggested by David Scott. In 1934 Scott, who was conducting experiments on insulin in the Connaught Laboratories found that crystalline insulin contained zinc. Furthermore, insulin from which zinc had been removed did not recrystallise. Scott demonstrated that this also applied to the solution of injected insulin. Interestingly the Lilly insulin was too pure and did not contain enough of the natural zinc of the pancreas.

In 1938 "crystalline insulin" was made available for sale in the United States. Unlike the two other types of insulin which were available commercially at the time namely, "regular"insulin and insulin with protamine and zinc (PZI), the rapidity with which the crystalline preparation started to act as well as the duration of its effect were unclear in the early stages of its use in the treatment of diabetes.

Crystallisation of insulin has a role in the practical treatment of diabetes in the modern era. Insulin analogues like lispro ("humalog") and aspart (novolog) which are insulins which have been changed so that there is less crystal formation are absorbed more quickly. When crystallisation is reduced in insulin preparations, their rapid absorption allows them to act more quickly.

A practical point stressed on today's patients with diabetes is that if the insulin looks cloudy it has become so because of crystals and will absorb less quickly then when the solution is clear. The practical advice given to patients with diabetes is that if the solution in the bottle from which the insulin is taken for daily injection changes its appearance in anyway the bottle has to be discarded.

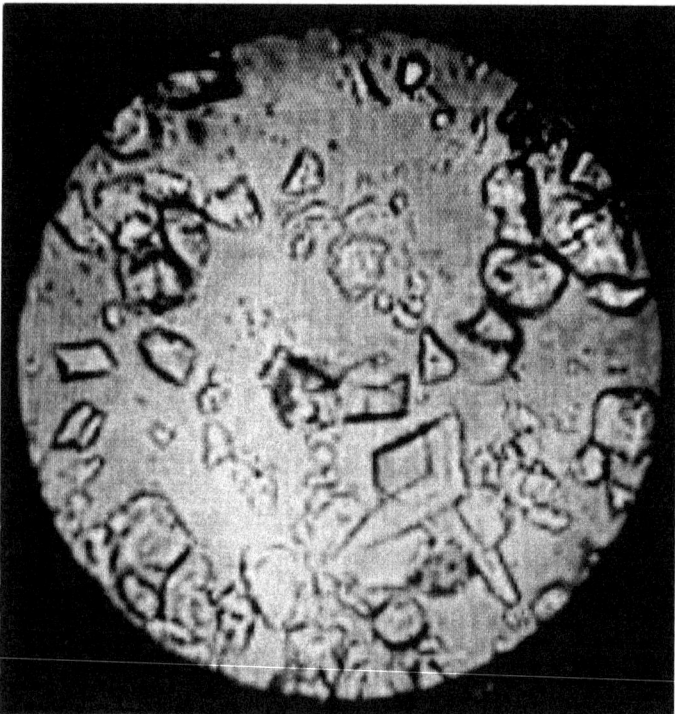

Insulin crystals

Collip's "lapse" perhaps not so "strange"

As a point of historical interest, the reader will not have failed to notice the parallel between Abel's temporary lapse in 1926-27 in producing crystalline insulin and Collip's failure in 1922 to reproduce his previously effective insulin extract for the treatment of diabetes following its initial success in Toronto. Banting had been convinced that Collip was not telling the truth and much was made of this including Michael Bliss's colourful account of a confrontation with Banting applying a headlock on the hapless Collip while Best helped by blocking the doorway to stop the biochemist escaping from his attacker ! (At least that was Best's version which he related many years later to Sir Henry Dale.)

I had also commented on the lack of assistance by Macleod in the matter. Had Collip been unfairly judged by Banting and Best– and also by me?

The Insulin Molecule Takes Centre Stage

Abel was convinced that the study of molecules and atoms held as much promise as the study of tissues and organs had held in earlier times through light microscopy. This had been recognised and emphasised by the earlier fathers of scientific thought and studies. One of the leading lights of European scientific community of relevance in the insulin story was the highly respected Rudolph Virchow (1821-1902), who had taught Paul Langerhans. Virchow impressed on his students the importance of using the microscope, often exhorting them to "think microscopically." The microscopic studies of sections of the pancreas by Langerhans for his thesis had first revealed the nests of the previously unrecognised cells which have guaranteed the medical student a permanent place in the history of diabetes, even in the history of medical advances.

John Jacob Abel may well have said, "think through molecules."

Known for his brilliance as a teacher not only because of his encyclopaedic knowledge but just as much, if not more, for his humility and modesty as a man, Abel remains a largely forgotten voice in most accounts of the history of progress in the knowledge and understanding of diabetes and also in the records of progress in the understanding of the chemistry of proteins including insulin.

(Virchow was also a popular left–wing politician in the German parliament at the time of the "Iron Chancellor" Otto von Bismarck (1815-1898). The story goes that the Conservative chancellor had been infuriated by Virchow and challenged him to a duel. According to the rules, the choice of weapon belongs to the recipient of the challenge, in this case, Virchow.

The Chancellor was infuriated when informed that the professor had chosen two pork sausages as weapons, with one of them inoculated with a deadly strain of bacteria. Virchow had informed the chancellor's messenger that the politician had first choice of the sausage! The Chancellor withdrew his challenge.

Whether the story is true or the product of a newsman's imagination poses a question which has never been answered.)

Looking Inside Insulin

> *"It is tempting to write the history of technology through products: the wheel; the microscope; the airplane; the Internet. But it is more illuminating to write the history of technology through transitions: linear motion to circular motion; visual space to subvisual space; motion on land to motion in the air; physical connectivity to virtual connectivity."*
> *– Siddhartha Mukherjee in The Gene An Intimate History.*

Refinement and improvement in insulin continued from its beginnings in Toronto in the summer of 1921. Changes achieved through technical advances reduced local reactions in the skin where the insulin was injected. The addition of zinc and protein prolonged the effect of an injection, a welcome respite from the need to inject themselves several times a day. Improvements in the methods of measuring glucose in the urine and later in the blood enable the patient to gauge more accurately the amount of insulin he needed to use.

However, the basic nature of insulin remained unchanged. It was sourced from the pancreas of animals – mainly cattle and pigs – and large quantities of pancreas were needed to produce only small amounts of insulin. One published estimate was that more than two tons of pig pancreases were needed to produce just eight ounces of purified insulin –"a near medieval method" – spat a modern researcher. Admittedly, this had not changed since the early times of Banting and Best.

Modern Insulin a Short History

The story of the discovery of Insulin as related earlier in this work shows interesting parallels but at the same time, marked contrasts with the story and understanding of the hormone as manufactured and used today. The history of the scientific pursuits by the Toronto researchers in 1921-22 is dominated by the small team of researchers namely Banting, Best, Collip and Macleod. Banting had had very little experience in medical research and Best was a student. Macleod at this stage was no longer active in research. Collip was a visiting Fellow for one summer.

A mere glance at the teams of scientists involved in the unravelling of the structure of insulin, as we have come to know in recent times, quickly reveals the differences between them and the Toronto team. The explosion in knowledge has inevitably resulted in greater degrees of specialisation. As a result the number of researchers in teams working on a project like insulin was predictably larger.

Prominent scientists in the modern insulin story include highly trained graduates and experienced researchers. The particular forte of each scientist is another indicator of the wide range of talented men and women who have contributed to different aspects of research into, and knowledge of, insulin as we know it today. The following (incomplete) list is in alphabetical order.

Oswald Avery – bacteriologist and geneticist
Paul Berg – biochemist
Herb Boyer– microbiologist

Stanley Cohen – microbial genetics
David Goeddell – chemist specialising in DNA
Frederick Griffith – bacteriologist
Dorothy Hodgkin – chemist
Keiichi Itakura – chemist specialising in DNA
Art Riggs – chemist specialising in DNA
Frederick Sanger – biochemist
Robert Swanson –venture capitalist
Rosalyn Yalow – physicist

Even an incomplete list as I have provided here shows that the larger number of scientists involved is largely because of greater specialisation in the various branches of science. The list is compiled from the teams in the United States. Similar teams worked in other countries and other centres including those in Britain, Germany and France. Various workers who were involved in developing insulin in Scandinavia have already been mentioned.

The much publicised Nobel Prize of 1923 for the discovery of insulin must be seen in a different context from the several Nobel prizes awarded to men and women in the modern history of research in several scientific fields including the unravelling of the insulin molecule.

As far as the Nobel Prize being awarded specifically for research on insulin, only the 1923 winners, Frederick Banting and James Macleod, still hold that particular distinction. Frederick Sanger could be included on the basis of the award being awarded for his work on "the structure of proteins especially insulin."

The research of several other Nobel Prize winners contributed significantly to the understanding and development of insulin.

Nobel Prize Winners in the Modern Insulin Story
Frederick Banting and James Macleod: 1923 Nobel Prize in Physiology or Medicine for discovering insulin.

Bernado Houssay: 1947 Nobel Prize in Physiology or Medicine for the relationship of the pituitary gland to glucose metabolism.

Frederick Sanger: 1958 Nobel prize in chemistry "for his work on the structure of proteins, especially insulin."

Frederick Sanger: 1980 jointly with Walter Gilbert for "contributions concerning the determination of the base sequences in nucleic acids."

Dorothy Crowfoot Hodgkin: 1964 Nobel Prize in chemistry for crystallography. Her work on insulin was done after the award.

Rosalyn Sussman Yalow: 1977 Nobel Prize in physiology or medicine for pioneering radioimmunoassay.

(Used by Donald Steiner to discover Proinsulin).

Paul Berg: 1980 Nobel Prize for chemistry for his gene splicing experiments which led to bacteria producing human insulin.

The Emergence of Modern Insulin

Around the time Frederick Banting was serving in the 1914-18 war, another Fredrick, an Englishman, was working at the Pathological Laboratories of the Ministry of Health which at that time were situated in London some 3 miles from the river Thames. That project was to prove pivotal in the development of modern insulin.

Frederick Griffith (1877–1941) was a medical graduate who had been employed by the British Ministry of Health in the early 1920s. He was born in England and was an alumnus of Liverpool University. His medical career had begun at the Liverpool Royal infirmary and continued in the Royal Commission on Tuberculosis. Like Banting, Griffith was also engaged in the war effort but did not see active duty. Apart from the role of each in the story there is little in common between the Canadian and the diminutive Englishman.

Griffith lived alone. He had a small house in Brighton but much of his time was spent in a small apartment situated close to the laboratory where he worked.

The government-funded laboratory where Griffith worked was taken over by the national government and became the Ministry of Health Bacteriological Laboratory. Griffiths was appointed as its medical officer. The National Government allocated minimal funding. However the bacteriologist was known for his resourcefulness and thrift. It was said that Griffith "could do more with a kerosene tin and a primus than most men could do with a palace."

At that time the bacteriologist, already with a reputation as a specialist in infection caused by germs, was studying the "pneumococcus". These bacteria which had caused the Spanish flu of 1918 had killed some 20 million men and women around the world.

Records show that death from pneumonia during the epidemic killed more men and women in the Armed Forces than the war itself. Once a patient had the flu he became susceptible to pneumococcus, rapidly developed pneumonia and nearly always lost his life soon afterwards. The devastating effects of this epidemic had caused the Ministry of Health to harness a team of scientists to find a vaccine to control the fatal disease.

Starting with a large number of samples of pneumococci taken from patients suffering from pneumonia, Griffith with this abundance of data started with searching for patterns of pneumonia as is done in epidemiology. He experimented on mice to gain an understanding of the pathology of pneumococcal pneumonia.

His capacity for working long hours combined with his capabilities as a scientist reminded me of the punishing schedule followed by Francis Madison Allen of diabetes fame described earlier in the insulin story. Another point of similarity between these two men was the very large number of experiments conducted by each one; Griffith on mice in the study of pneumonia, and Allen on dogs and other animals in his work on pancreatic diabetes.

Griffith's critical discovery was the transfer of genetic material between unrelated bacteria.

This phenomenon of transferring the characteristics or attributes from one type of bacteria to another unrelated type is referred to, in scientific jargon as *transformation*. Remarkably, Griffiths had discovered this in the early 1920s when the chemistry of living organisms was in its infancy.

Unlike the assertive Canadian Frederick Banting, Griffiths, as described by the Pulitzer Prize–winning writer Siddhartha Mukherjee in his captivating account of the current understanding of genetics in *The Gene, An Intimate History* (Simon & Schuster 2016), was "an unassuming, painfully shy scientist – this tiny man who… barely spoke in a whisper"– could hardly be expected to broadcast the broader relevance or appeal of his results."

Griffith's experiment, in essence, consisted of working with two strands of pneumococcus; one strain which had a smooth coat he called the "smooth strain." This was the lethal strain. The second strain of pneumococcus was different in that it lacked the smooth coat. Griffith called this the rough strain. The rough strain had no ill effects.

The Man Who Launched the Molecular Biology Revolution

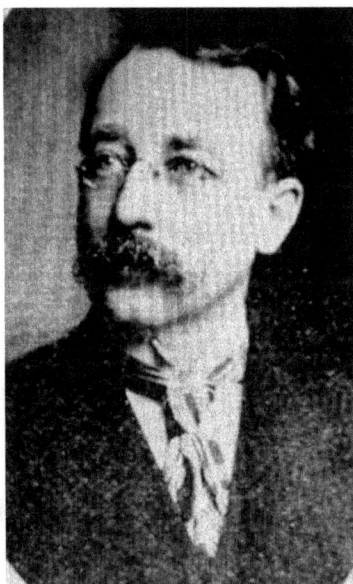

Frederick Griffith pioneered molecular chemistry.

Fred Griffith's experiment which, Mukherjee says, "launched the molecular biology revolution" consisted of four simple steps.

First, Griffiths killed the infected smooth strain with heat and injected the material into mice. The injections had no effect.

Secondly, he combined the material of the dead strain (which was no longer lethal), with the second "rough" strain which had been harmless on its own.

Thirdly, after mixing the dead smooth strain, with the rough strain, he injected the mixture into mice. The mice died.

Finally, Griffith examined the dead mice and made the astounding discovery that the "rough strain" pneumococcus had actually changed to the "smooth strain" variety.

He concluded that contact with material from the death – causing smooth strain had changed the harmless rough strain pneumococcus to the lethal smooth strain variety.

The experiment revealed that the dead material from the smooth strain, although in itself harmless when killed by heat, could by simply being in contact with the hitherto harmless "rough strain" change the latter into the smooth strain, lethal pneumococcus.

Griffith's work showed that through the process now called *transformation*, genetic material could be transmitted from one organism (in this case one kind of pneumococcus) to another without any active reproduction. Thus, genes could carry – and spread – information from organism to unrelated organism.

It was this principle of "transformation" defined then developed and refined which eventually led to the use of E. coli, a common bacterial organism to produce insulin.

Griffith published his findings in the *Journal of Hygiene, Volume 27, 113–159 in 1928* under the title, *The Significance of Pneumococcal Types.*

The article detailed his experiments on the basis of which Griffith stated that he had "manipulated the immunologic specificity in pneumococci."

His claim left the scientific world stunned and speechless.

At that time the chemistry of living organisms was in the very early stages of scientific enquiry. There had not been any concerted efforts at studying it. Yet here was an unknown bacteriologist claiming that he not only could but actually had manipulated a hitherto untouched fundamental biological phenomenon.

At the time the effect of Griffith's discovery on modern molecular chemistry and the eventual "cracking of the code" through his work on "transformation" was regarded by many as the first step which culminated in the synthesis of insulin several decades later.

Griffith by nature was self-effacing. He eschewed publicity and never sought the limelight But his claim was bound to give him prominence in scientific circles of that time. And beyond.

It was no surprise that Griffith's experiments had attracted attention of a man whose efforts were to write the next chapter in the story begun by the Englishman. His name was Oswald Avery.

Oswald Avery (1877–1955) Interpreter of Dreams. Avery, like Banting, was a Canadian. He was born in Halifax, Nova Scotia and had a protestant background. His father Joseph Avery was a Baptist minister who had emigrated from Britain in 1873. Christian teachings remained a lifelong influence on young Oswald. In 1887, the 10-year-old moved with the family as an immigrant to the United States and settled in New York City where he was to spend the next 60 years.

Although Avery spent most of his working life in the United States, the small timber row-house on Marine Street in the north end of Halifax is now a designated heritage building.

Avery's family moved to the lower east side of New York City when he was 10 years old. Although his early interest was in music he switched to Medicine at college and graduated in 1904. After devoting three years to a practice in general surgery he turned to research.

Rufus Cole, Director of the Rockefeller Institute Hospital recognised Avery's uncanny analytical capabilities and appointed him to the hospital in 1913. Avery spent the rest of his life there.

Thus while Banting was serving on the front in 1918–1919, Avery was part of the research team at the Rockefeller Institute in New York which developed the first effective immune serum against a strain of pneumococcus which causes pneumonia.

Avery was an extremely private man. He never divulged details of his personal life to anyone including his colleagues. He once said that he believed that knowledge of matters unrelated to a scientist's work in the laboratory should have no bearing on the valuation or understanding of his scientific accomplishment.

At the time of Griffith's announcement Avery was away from the laboratory because of severe Graves' disease, a condition caused by an over-active thyroid gland. Given his nature, Avery was not impressed with Griffith's claim which he considered was rather grandiose. He pointed to parts of the bacteriologist's work which he considered showed inadequate experimental design.

Perhaps a deeply religious Avery was affronted by what he considered a lack of humility in Griffith. However he did not persist with his criticism but changed his own focus to study the transmissible hereditary changes revealed in Griffith's experiments.

It is part of history that Avery produced the next milestone in this branch of biology.

At first Avery repeated Griffith's experiments and like Griffith found that the smooth coated bacteria after being "transformed" had become virulent. This was in the spring of 1940, twelve years after the publication of Griffith's findings.

But Avery went a step further.

His team of three which included two assistants, Colin McLeod and Maclyn McCarty embarked on the painstaking task of separating the bacterial elements to identify the actual substance of the transforming principle which transmitted the genetic information.

The end result of this painstaking experiment was Avery's realisation that the transforming principle was in fact DNA.

In other words, DNA carried out the "transformation" described by Griffiths.

Avery realised the implications of the finding and called it "something that has long been the dream of geneticists*".

In fact he was hesitant, perhaps even afraid, to publish his findings which he did in 1944.

His experiments showed conclusively that the substance responsible for transferring genetic information (ie Griffith's transforming principle), was in fact Desoxyribonucleic acid better known as DNA. Genes were actually made of DNA.

Oswald Avery published his findings on DNA in1944.

Although clearly aware of the implications of his discovery, given his natural tendency to caution, Avery was hesitant to make any grandiose claims or announcements.

Others were not as reticent.

Peter Brian Medawar, (later Sir Peter), known for his facility with English vocabulary and phraseology praised Avery's discovery as "the first step out of the dark ages of genetics."

Simply put, Griffith's work, repeated and confirmed by Avery showed that DNA which contained genetic material in the form of genes was accessible. After all, boiling the bacteria as Avery had done still allowed genetic material to be taken from one bacterial strain to another "transformed" the recipient. This simple but hitherto unexplored development–perhaps because its possibilities had not been fully appreciated – was to play a critical part in a dramatic new development in the production of insulin.

---

* The deeply religious Avery brought up by strict Baptist parents may have regretted referring to his work as a dream, remembering the biblical reference to the interpretation of dreams in the story of Joseph who interpreted the dreams of the Pharaoh.

Some regard Avery's discovery as the single most important advance in that field (biology) in the 20th century.

However, hand-in-hand with the potential for dramatic new development came concerns of an ethical nature in the event of unexpected results of transferring genetic material from one class of say, viruses or bacteria to another such as animals – or humans.

These possibilities which troubled many of the workers in this field, among them one of the leading researchers, Paul Berg will be addressed later in this account.

Griffith's experiments repeated by Avery led to the next leap in unlocking one of the great mysteries of biology by the much-publicised* work of the Cambridge duo, Francis Crick and James Watson. In fact DNA had been identified much earlier. In 1869 the Swiss physiologist and chemist Friederich Miescher had identified what he called "nuclein" (later called nucleic acid) inside the nuclei of human white blood cells.

Not that the two young men especially Francis Crick needed anyone else to publicise their work. I have read more than one account of Crick walking into The Eagle, (a pub in Cambridge owned by the Corpus Christi College of the University of Cambridge which dates its beginnings from 1667), at lunchtime on 28th of February 1953 to declare (in his booming voice) that he and James Watson had "discovered the secret of life" referring to their proposal for the structure of DNA.

Author's apology

In my preparations for this book on insulin it was difficult to leave the early groundbreaking research on DNA dominated by scientists of extraordinary brilliance.

However "I have promises to keep…" and must return to the story of insulin.

So we leave the stories of remarkable men like Linus Pauling and Francis Crick and James Watson.

But do not despair. You will now meet more men and women of great accomplishment and charisma as we embark on the final part of this narrative which leads to insulin as it is used today.

Crystallography

Many of the facts that have come to light might well be the subject of lectures adapted to a juvenile auditory, and would be at the same time interesting and helpful; interesting because they display a beautiful order in the fundamental arrangement of nature, and helpful because they have given us light on many old questions, and will surely help us with many that are new.
Sir William Henry Bragg. 1927.

Sydney Brenner (1927–2019), the South African biologist and the 2002 Nobel Laureate in Physiology or Medicine who had made significant contributions to molecular biology maintained that progress in science depended on new techniques, new discoveries and new ideas. Then, perhaps to be provocative as was his nature, he added "probably in that order."

The three-dimensional double helix described and demonstrated by the Cambridge researchers owed a considerable debt to a new tool of investigation called X-ray crystallography which overcame to a large extent two challenges for investigative molecular chemists in the early years. The first was to overcome the difficulty in understanding the minuteness of the scale of action and properties of atoms and the second to understand this new entity as it existed in space.

Crystallography, by which crystalline atoms cause a beam of x-ray to deflect into many specific directions, allows scientists to determine the make-up of a particular crystal.

The 22-year-old William Lawrence Bragg, a pioneer in this field, and the son of Sir William Henry Bragg had a special connection with Australia because he was born in Adelaide and where at that time his father, at the age of 23, had been appointed Professor of Mathematics and Experimental Physics at the University of Adelaide. William Bragg had graduated from Cambridge University the previous year at the age of 22 with a first class honours degree in mathematics.

The older Bragg, had developed a particular interest in the field of electromagnetism from an early age. He had been fascinated by a discovery described in a hobby–magazine by a German called William Roentgen.

In 1896 in Adelaide, Bragg demonstrated before a meeting of local general practitioners the application of "x-rays to reveal structures that were otherwise invisible." A chemist from the well-known Adelaide pharmaceutical company of F.H. Faulding & Co. had supplied a glass tube known as Crookes tube which he had obtained from Leeds in England when visiting a manufacturer of photographic and laboratory equipment. Using these rudimentary pieces Bragg impressed his audience of local doctors especially when he allowed his hand to be "x-rayed"and even more when the image showed an old injury in one of his fingers.

Bragg recalled the incident which he said had occurred many years earlier when he had been helping on his father's farm in Cumbria.

Another "x-ray" story is about young Lawrence Bragg who shortly after starting school had an accident when riding his tricycle and broke his arm. Sir William, using his home-made equipment which employed x-rays as described by Roentgen, made the correct diagnosis of a fracture in his son's forearm. This is said to have been the first recorded surgical use of x-rays in Australia.

The most concise description of crystallography is provided by the younger Bragg, William Lawrence, who stated that the essence of crystallography was x-ray diffraction by a crystal (which arose from the reflection of the x-rays) by planes of atoms in the crystal.

Both father and son, Sir William and Sir Lawrence Bragg are considered the pioneers of crystallography.

They also hold the unique honour of a father and son sharing the Nobel Prize for Physics which was awarded in 1915 "for their services in the analysis of crystal structures by means of x-rays."

The use of crystallography in the last hundred years has transformed the understanding of various phenomena in chemistry, meteorology, and recently, biology.

The relevance of crystallography in the insulin story lies in its use in elucidating the structure of insulin and facilitating investigations pertinent to insulin.

The description of crystallography and its critical role in providing further insight into the structure of insulin is a good time in this narrative to introduce some remarkable women whose contributions led to a greater understanding of insulin structure and function.

The obstacles and barriers which women had to overcome at the very first stage of any significant academic (and social) advancement are part of the social history of many cultures. Unfortunately many barriers to the advancement of women persist even in today's so called enlightened world.

THREE REMARKABLE WOMEN IN THE HISTORY OF MODERN INSULIN

Dorothy Hodgkin, Crystallography's Leading Lady (1910-1994)

"There was magic about her person ...like the spring."
Max Perutz, Nobel Prize winning crystallographer

Dorothy Hodgkin was born Dorothy Mary Crowfoot in Cairo, Egypt where her father worked in Colonial Administration. Dorothy, as a child played with pebbles she found in a stream behind their home in Khartoum. Her father was also an archaeologist and encouraged his daughter's interest in stones.

Dorothy's mother gave her a gift of a book written by Sir William Bragg which explained in simple language the complexities of object like stones. The mathematics professor who was later recognised and honoured as a pioneer of crystallography would never have known that a child fascinated by his book would one day win the Nobel Prize for research carried out using the technique he had given to science.

The highly respected and multi-talented Dorothy Hodgkin also had a social conscience and was active politically. She was never too busy to listen to issues which concerned or troubled her students. Many remained in contact with her even after leaving Oxford

University. One ex-student who consulted her from time to time even when she had gone into politics was Margaret Thatcher.

In addition to her work in the laboratory and in social circles, Hodgkin was also a committed activist. Her mother's four brothers were killed during the Second World War. In her Anti-war effort she was often in contact with Linus Pauling another Nobel Laureate (Chemistry) who was awarded a second Nobel Prize, (for Peace) for his campaigns against nuclear weapons.

Hodgkin was well ahead of her time in multitasking which included raising three children, tutoring students, supporting her busy husband and still finding time to advise her students in coping with academic challenges as well as personal difficulties. At the same time she herself had suffered from crippling arthritis from her late 20s. Even during her period of scientific achievements it was a battle for her to get up and get dressed in the morning. "Every joint in my body seemed to be affected," she said.

She had followed in the footsteps of an earlier luminary in the insulin story. John Jacob Abel had published his method for obtaining the rhombohedral crystals of insulin. Unlike Hodgkin however, Abel received little praise or recognition for his seminal contribution, let alone the Nobel Prize.

Hodgkin's method of positioning the crystals for her studies is still used today. The technique which she had devised enabled her to reveal the details of the structure of crystals more clearly than any workers who had attempted this exercise previously.

Her accomplishments with crystallography won Hodgkin the Nobel Prize for Chemistry in 1964.

Her work on insulin crystals in the mid 1950s was given further impetus by Frederick Sanger whose discovery of the exact order, (*sequence*) of the building blocks of insulin stimulated Hodgkin to work on the crystal structure of the hormone. Whereas Sanger was assiduously pursuing his goal of identifying the exact sequence of the building blocks of proteins, Hodgkin's interest was in the three-dimensional shape taken on by proteins. Here she struck a stumbling block. When she looked at Insulin she realised that by comparison with other structures insulin was a molecule of daunting size. Its complexity made it extremely difficult, almost impossible to get a clear image.

Determined to work in the same field, Hodgkin switched to two smaller molecules. She started by studying penicillin with which she helped the war effort by producing more refined preparations of the antibiotic. Then it was vitamin B12. Although these were smaller molecules than insulin the work required long hours and meticulous attention to detail. It took her four years to demonstrate the three-dimensional form of penicillin and eight years to achieve the same goal for vitamin B12.

In 1969, 34 years after her earlier studies on insulin, Hodgkin returned to the project. Her work with insulin helped its mass production, an essential pre-requisite for supplying diabetics whose daily need for Insulin injections was dependent on its availability.

Rosalyn Sussman Yalow and Radioimmunoassay

"From the typing pool to the Nobel Prize for Physics"

Roslyn Yalow was an American medical physicist and Nobel Laureate for Physiology or Medicine 1977.

The Centennial of the discovery of insulin in the summer of 1921 coincided with another event in that same summer which was destined to occupy a place of distinction in the insulin story albeit some years later.

It is the story of Rosalyn Sussman Yalow (1921–2011). Yalow was born on July 19, 1921 in a poor Jewish household in the Bronx, New York.

She received much of her education in tuition-free schools. She taught herself to type and secured a part-time secretarial position at Columbia University's College of Physicians and Surgeons hoping to gain entry into a Science course but left when she realised that the graduate school would not admit a woman. She was employed by a biochemist who hired her on condition that she studied shorthand–typing. At that time most women believed that the only acceptable path for a woman in science was to become a high school science teacher.

When the Second World War broke out in 1939 and many men enlisted, the university began to offer places to women so as to avoid being shut down. Yalow was the only woman in the University of Illinois' 400 members and the first since 1917. Even after earning a PhD in 1945 at the age of 24 years she still sought tuition-free courses in physics offered by the government at New York University.

After her marriage to a rabbi's son in 1943, she faithfully kept a "kosher" home, never questioning the traditional domestic roles including those of motherhood. Yalow shunned feminist organisations but at the same time remained a steadfast advocate for "women in science".

In her acceptance speech at the Nobel ceremony, Yalow said, "The world cannot afford the loss of the talents of half its people if we are to solve the many problems which beset us."

The era of radioimmunoassay began in 1959. It was the result of a collaborative effort between Roslyn Yalow and Solomon Berson who worked together at the Bronx Veterans Administration Hospital in New York from 1950 to Berson's death in 1972.

The extreme sensitivity of this method allows minute quantities of blood to be analysed to determine the concentration of different substances in it.

In the case of insulin, radioimmunoassay permits the detection of even infinitesimal amounts of insulin present in a given sample. The use of the method lends itself to the measurement of antibodies to various agents including viruses which cause hepatitis.

The technical details of radioimmunoassay (RA) were reported in the prestigious Journal of Clinical Investigation (JCI) in 1956. It was Yalow's most significant contribution to medicine – a discovery she made together with her colleague Solomon Berson.

This method made it possible to measure the presence of hormones in the blood in concentrations as low as 1000 billionth of a gram per millilitre of blood. Since many hormones in the human body are present in the blood in such small quantities the usefulness of this technique requires no emphasis. Before Yalow's discovery these hormones could not be determined quantitatively in the blood. As a result research in this field had stagnated.

Yalow was awarded the Nobel Prize for Physiology or Medicine in 1977. Unfortunately Solomon Berson had died some years earlier and therefore was not eligible to share the award. Yalow never forgot the contribution Bersen had made to her research and her life.

Radioimmunoassay continues to occupy an important position as an irreplaceable instrument in scientific investigation.

At the Nobel presentation ceremony, Rolf Luft of the Karolinska Institute declared that, "the Yalow – Berson method represents a real revolution in the field of hormone research. Her methodology and the modifications thereof subsequently made the triumphant journey far beyond her own field of research, reaching into vast territories of biology and medicine."

An important consequence from the point of view of this account on the discovery of Insulin is that in 1967 Donald Steiner (1930–2014) using radioimmunoassay discovered that human Insulin was produced as a single chain which Steiner called *proinsulin.*

Of greater consequence perhaps was that this discovery increased the understanding of hormone production in general.

The discovery of details of the structure of insulin as well as how it works in those suffering from diabetes owe much to these two techniques namely, radioimmunoassay and crystallography.

Birte Marie Krogh (1874–1943)

I learned a great deal about Marie and August Krogh from reading an excellent biography, *August and Marie Krogh Lives in Science.* It was written by their daughter, herself a distinguished physiologist, Dr. Bodil Schmidt-Nielsen.

Like the other two women mentioned previously, Marie Krogh had suffered hardships before becoming part of the insulin story. She was born into the Jorgensen family on Christmas Day 1874. Of the nine children in the family she was one of only four who survived into adulthood.

Owing to difficulties including poverty in her family Marie had to delay her education and finally embarked on her university course in 1901 at the age of 27. At university she had met and married August Krogh, the future Nobel Laureate in Physiology. August Krogh was the son of a brewer. He had studied zoology in Copenhagen, earning his doctorate under the guidance of the physiologist Christian Bohr.

Marie Krogh graduated in medicine in 1907 at the age of 33. She went into medical practice to supplement their far from adequate joint incomes. Her husband was spending all his time on medical research which unfortunately, like research even today, does not attract any more than minimal funding.

In 1907 Marie became the fourth woman in Denmark to earn a medical doctorate which that time was unusual especially for a married woman.

In her practice she treated a number of children with diabetes.

She herself had developed diabetes during the early 1920s. She and her husband had heard a great deal about the research on insulin during their visit to the United States and Canada in 1922.

August Krogh had been awarded the Nobel Prize for Physiology or Medicine for his work on the blood flow in capillaries during exercise.

In the fall of 1922 he went on an extensive lecture tour in the United States the highlight of which was the Silliman Lecture at Yale University.

Krogh and his wife had travelled by ship to the United States. When they visited Boston in early October they met Elliott Joslin, already well known in Europe as an expert on diabetes largely because of his reputation for treating a large number of patients with diabetes as well as his textbook on the subject published in 1916.

At a private dinner Joslin told Marie Krogh about the discovery, development and purification of insulin in Toronto and described in detail the dramatic effects of insulin on his patients. She was aware of the arrangement between Toronto and the Medical Research Council in England to facilitate insulin production there.

Joslin suggested to Marie Krogh that just as doctors in America had received doses of the insulin extract from Toronto perhaps she could also get some of the newly discovered potion.

It was following her suggestion that her husband wrote to a fellow-physiologist in Toronto University called James Macleod. James Macleod was only too willing to welcome the new Nobel Laureate as a houseguest as detailed elsewhere in this story.

Marie Krogh's story also includes her professional association with a young Danish physician called Hans Christian Hagedorn had developed a special interest in treating diabetes. The two had met at a medical conference and become friends.

In 1918 Hagedorn had worked with a local pharmacist and developed a method for determining blood sugar levels which required very small samples of blood which could be drawn from a needle prick in the earlobe. Hagedorn had done his PhD thesis on blood sugar regulation. He had also written a paper on the Allen – Joslin diet treatment of diabetes.

In 1921 or early 1922 Hagedorn had diagnosed Marie Krogh's Diabetes (type 2 also called adult-onset diabetes, which did not need insulin for treatment).

Like many who suffered from any chronic ailment at that time, Marie Krogh had kept her condition a secret from all beyond her immediate family.

However it was Marie Krogh's suggestion that resulted in getting permission from the Toronto workers for insulin to be manufactured in Denmark. That was the beginning of the Novo Insulin production in Denmark.

The second important contribution Marie Krogh made to the development of insulin was to encourage Hagedorn to look at the new preparation from Toronto "from a theoretical as well as a practical point of view."

She also told Hagedorn, "Since I believe you will be interested in this preparation, I have persuaded my husband to write to Dr MacLeod in Toronto and ask him if it is possible to get the production method so that it would be possible for you to make experiments with the preparation in Denmark."

Marie Krogh had guessed correctly.

Hagedorn liked the idea.

He stopped practising medicine and eagerly welcomed the Kroghs on their return to Copenhagen in late autumn 1922.

The very next day, after discussing the project with August Krogh, Hagedorn decided to start on research to produce insulin. He worked in a laboratory which had been built in his home.

In Marie Krogh's correspondence on insulin there is no reference to her own diabetes.

Nor is there any mention of Banting and Best.

I found online a copy of the handwritten letter by August Krogh to Professor Mac Leod (*sic*).

August Krogh wrote to Macleod on October 23, 1922 telling him about his forthcoming trip to the United States and his lecture tour and said "I have been hearing everywhere about the experimental treatment of diabetes with insulin and I have been wondering if perhaps it might be consistent with the plan of yourself and your collaborators to have experiments carried out in Denmark also."

Probably unaware of Macleod's own interest and background in carbohydrate metabolism, Krogh assured him that Hagedorn was "a very competent investigator and specialist in diabetes. He has done some very good work which unfortunately so far has only been published in Danish. He has worked out and thoroughly tested a new micro method for blood sugar determination, which I think is the best in existence."

Krogh also said that Hagedorn "would be able to do very good work with the insulin and I would, of course be willing to undertake any supervision which you might desire."

Whether Krogh had heard about the difficulties with the preparation of the extract because of the limited experience of both Banting and Best in laboratory bench–work, is not known. One could speculate that given Elliott Joslin's avid interest in research relating to insulin, he may well have passed that on to the Kroghs at the time he had told Marie Krogh of the discovery in Toronto. This would explain Krogh telling Macleod that he had in his laboratory "at least one organic chemist with considerable experience in preparative work who would be able and willing to undertake the preparation of insulin for our own use, if you would give us the necessary directions."

Krogh confidently stated that "the pancreas material and the money would, I have reason to believe, be easily obtainable in Denmark." He was of course referring to bacon, a national favourite breakfast staple produced by a thriving industry devoted to pork. Consequently there was a plentiful supply of pancreases from slaughtered pigs.

Krogh accepted Macleod's invitation for them to stay with him and his wife as house guests after lecturing in Cleveland. Krogh ended his letter with "I do hope that it will be found possible to extend to Denmark the privilege of taking part in the work of delivering this wonderful new discovery." Clearly his wife had told him about the "privilege" the Torontonians had extended to their British cousins.

Macleod, was clearly delighted to have the Nobel Laureate as a house guest. The visit was arranged for November 23–25. He wrote back saying "to have your department take up some work on insulin, particularly since it will be put in charge of Dr Hagedorn, with whose work, of course, I am familiar. I should like very much to go over our insulin work with you and get the benefit of your advice and cooperation. The Kroghs, both husband and wife, spent considerable time in meetings with

Macleod and Banting and left Toronto with formal authorisation from the University of Toronto Insulin committee to introduce insulin to Scandinavia.

It was Marie Krogh who persuaded him to remain involved in working on insulin. It is a matter of historical record that her role in initially establishing contact in Toronto as well as involving Hagedorn in the work on insulin was of great importance in the development of insulin in Europe. Later insulin was produced and marketed in other European countries especially Germany and France.

Once back in Denmark, the close cooperation between Hagedorn and Krogh ultimately resulted in the production of insulin in that country as outlined in this account.

Marie Krogh developed breast cancer and died in 1943.

Her influence pioneered the development of insulin in Denmark but perhaps of greater significance in the insulin story is the role she played in involving Hans Christian Hagedorn in the development of insulin which resulted in the breakthrough preparation of Protamine Zinc Insulin by Hagedorn which relieved patients of the burden of having several injections each day.

Hagedorn remained involved in the development and marketing of insulin for the rest of his life.

Insulin Unravelled

"Your sons and daughters will prophesy, your old men will dream dreams, your young men will see visions."

Joel. (an Israeli prophet.)

FREDERICK SANGER THE SHY GENIUS WHO UNRAVELLED INSULIN

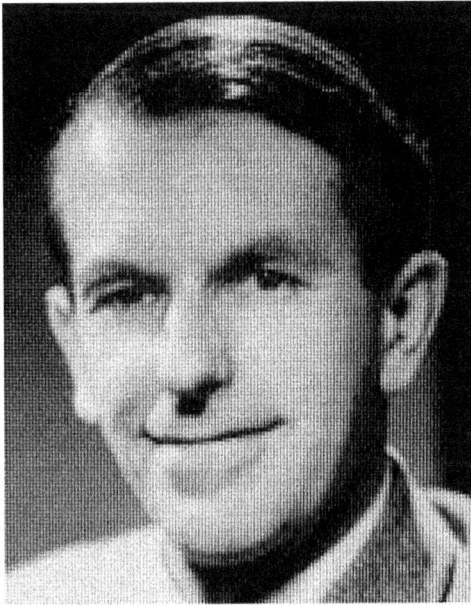

Frederick Sanger looked inside insulin.

Sanger was born in Rendcomb, a small village in Gloucestershire, England on August 13, 1918. His father, Frederick Sanger was a general practitioner. Sanger's mother Cicely Sanger (née Crewdson) was the daughter of a wealthy cotton merchant. His father had served in China as a medical missionary but on his return had adopted the practices of Quakerism, a Protestant Christian denomination which avoids religious conventions and church hierarchy.

One of my university friends who was a Quaker took me to a Quaker "meeting" at which the congregation remained standing and silent for the entire duration of worship. There was no preaching or singing or prayer. He told me that that was a form of "waiting worship"and if one felt inclined to speak that was allowed but frequently the entire time was given to silent contemplation. Quakers place great emphasis on simplicity in their private lives and their dress codes. They refuse to swear oaths, forego all alcoholic beverages and remain firm in their opposition to war.

Sanger did not convert to Quakerism but remained opposed to war. Throughout his life he was ascetic in his conduct and habits. His conscientious–objector status was respected by the authorities and therefore he did not take part in the war effort.

Young Sanger's interest in chemistry was awakened early in his schooling as he went to a liberal school where he had spent the last year of his primary education experimenting in the chemistry laboratory alongside his chemistry master who himself had studied at Cambridge and had been a researcher in the Cavendish Laboratory.

In 1936 Sanger started at St John's College, Cambridge to study natural sciences. His father had attended the same college to study medicine.

Sanger was not a brilliant student. He had difficulty with physics and mathematics and in his second year, switched from physics to physiology. He excelled at biochemistry obtaining a first class honours in the subject.

Tragically during his first two years at Cambridge both his parents died, his father at 60 and his mother at 58. A substantial inheritance following his parents' death enabled Sanger to engage in research instead of becoming a teacher as he had planned because he did not have the financial resources to enable him to engage in research at Cambridge.

He chose to study science and obtained a doctorate with a thesis on the metabolism of the amino acid lysine.

In later years Sanger told one of his friends that he was not going to follow his father's footsteps and practise medicine because he saw his father "running around from problem to problem in different patients and never having time to solve anything complex."

In 1926, John Jacob Abel, the Head of Johns Hopkins' first Department of Pharmacology had shown that insulin was a protein. Proteins are made up of chains of amino acid.

When Sanger was studying biochemistry the knowledge of the structure of proteins was in its infancy. In 1943 he started working with a protein chemist at Cambridge called Albert Chibnall. Chibnall believed that proteins were distinct chemical compounds. As indicated earlier, the contributions of John Jacob Abel which had been reported in 1926 still had not gained widespread acceptance. It is unclear whether Chibnall or for that matter Sanger was familiar with the Johns Hopkins' pharmacologist's earlier contributions.

Chibnall himself had worked on the amino acid composition of bovine insulin.

He gave Sanger the assignment of identifying the composition of insulin. Unlike many other compounds for scientific use insulin, which had been discovered by Banting in Toronto 20 years earlier, was being produced in pure form by pharmaceutical companies all round the world for treatment of diabetics. One of the prominent retailers in Britain was the pharmacy chain of Boots Chemists. Supplies were therefore readily available for experimental studies. Working with bovine insulin, Sanger confirmed that proteins had a definite chemical composition, something which had been suggested by John Jacob Abel over 20 years earlier.

Sanger showed that insulin was composed of fifty-one basic units (amino acids) arranged in two chains. The A chain is made up of 21 amino acids and the B chain of 30 amino acids.

The two chains are held together with links between sulphur atoms (disulphide bonds). In 1952 and 1951 respectively, Sanger determined the complete amino acid sequence of the two polypeptide chains B and A of bovine insulin. After this he also had to determine the nature of the sulphur joining-pieces, "disulphide bonds" in scientific jargon, which joined the two chains because without these, the two chains of insulin were entirely inactive.

Sanger, by determining the actual sequence of the amino acids in the two chains demonstrated that proteins were made up of specific amino acids which were located at specific sites. The effect of a particular protein depends on the order (sequence) and details of the shape of its amino acids.

Sanger was the first scientist to demonstrate the "sequence" of a protein – in this case insulin. These experiments occupied Sanger working, as Mukherjee describes, "in a hutlike laboratory buried half-underground near the fens" for nearly 12 years. For this groundbreaking discovery he was awarded the Nobel Prize for Chemistry in 1958.

The fens, originally a marshy region occupying nearly 4000 km² which was drained and reclaimed centuries ago is situated in Cambridgeshire. In earlier times its monasteries attracted visitors. The Ely Cathedral is still a popular tourist attraction. In recent times the fens has also been used as an agricultural area but still needs to be protected from flooding.

Buildings in the area have to contend with dampness and there is little doubt that the working conditions for Sanger in his small laboratory would have been challenging. Little wonder that moving from this to the modern facilities in the summer of 1962 when he started in a laboratory in the Medical Research Council (MRC) building in Cambridge may well have given him a new lease of life.

According to Mukherjee, "The transition of labs marked a seminal transition in Sanger's focus."

Sanger's methods were of his own design. They were new and innovative and remain in use to this day.

A critical finding which alone would guarantee Sanger a place in the history of scientific achievements was his demonstration that like insulin, every protein has a unique sequence. This led to the "sequence hypothesis" which played an important role in Crick's and Watson's ideas on DNA codes for proteins.

Later workers in the field extended Sanger's methods which eventually led to automated protein sequencing. Modern instruments for automated protein sequencing can accomplish in days what previously took several years of labouring at the laboratory bench.

Today it is common practice to sequence proteins and cheaper and quicker methods of automated sequencing remain at the forefront of research in molecular chemistry.

(See postscript).

In 1987 Sanger became one of only two men to win a second Nobel prize in the same discipline when his work on genetic codes proved to be the first steps in the new science of *genomics,* a branch of biology concerned with the study of genes and the way genes react with other genes and also with the environment. (The other man to win two Nobel Prizes in the same discipline was John Bardeen for Physics.)

Although not directly related to the development of modern insulin, Sanger's work which began in 1962 at the Medical Research Council building in Cambridge introduced a new method for sequencing DNA molecules. The use of this method permitted long stretches of DNA to be rapidly and accurately sequenced and earned Sanger his second Nobel Prize in Chemistry in 1980 which he shared with Walter Gilbert and Paul Berg.

I have included this connection between Sanger and Berg because the latter played a critical role in the development of modern insulin.

It is thought provoking that Sanger, in addition to his brilliance as a scientist also possessed the often unrecognised character trait in many, if not most accomplished men and women namely, resilience and tenacity.

After his success with insulin, Sanger turned his hand to sequencing DNA and once again excelled himself. His second Nobel Prize in Chemistry in 1980, shared with Walter Gilbert and Paul Berg, came 22 years after his first Nobel. If as has been said, scientific research is an endurance sport, Sanger would qualify as a marathon runner. Little wonder that he is almost unique in winning two Nobel prizes in the same discipline.

The prestigious journal *Science* perhaps noted the most appropriate and admired quality of Fredrick Sanger's personality when it said that he was "the most self-effacing person you could hope to meet."

Shy and introverted, Sanger was also a man of few words. However he was aware of his prowess as a scientist. At a gathering of his colleagues after his second Nobel Prize had been announced and he had been praised, Sanger famously responded with,

"I want you all to know that I think that I am bloody good."

No one would begrudge this remarkable man a rare moment of levity.

Sanger retired in 1983 when he was 65 years old. He was honoured, respected and admired. When offered a knighthood he refused because "I don't want to be different."

He attributed his success to the love and devotion of his wife Margaret Joan Howe. She had died in 2012.

In 1986 Sanger accepted a rare honour, the Order of Merit which can have only 24 living members.

In 1992 the Wellcome Trust and the Medical Research Council founded the Sanger Centre now called the Sanger Institute. Sanger agreed to open the centre himself on for 4 October 1993. The centre is regarded as one of the world's leading establishments which played a role in the sequencing of the human genome.

Sanger died in his sleep in 2013 at the age of 95. In his obituary he stated that he was "academically not brilliant."

Insulin, Dissected, Divided and Diced

Sanger's groundbreaking research set in train a succession of transitions in the insulin molecule best described in the alliterative phrase used in the title. These transitions were achieved through the research carried out by several scientists and resulted in the making of modern insulin.

A Chain

B Chain

PAUL BERG (1926 –) MORE THAN A SCIENTIST

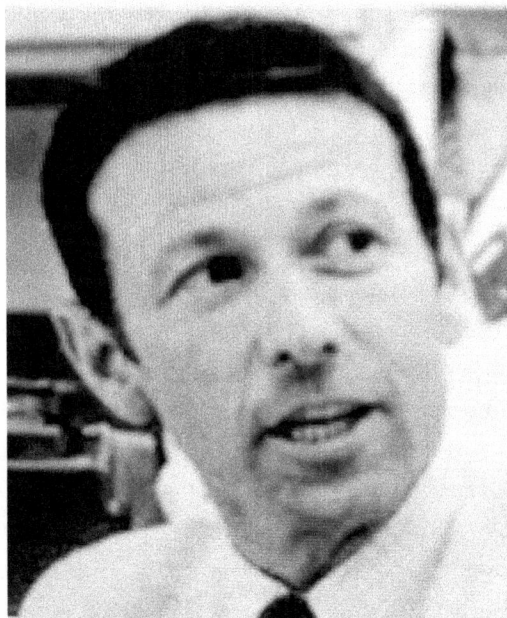

Paul Berg pioneered recombinant technology

One word commonly associated with modern insulin is "recombinant" and the name Paul Berg is often uttered in the same breath. Berg has the unique distinction of being the first investigator to build a recombinant DNA molecule. The recombinant nature of this molecule consisted of fragments of the chromosomes (which house the DNA) from unrelated and distinct species namely a viral and a bacterial chromosome. (Berg himself had coined the word).

For this Berg was awarded the Nobel Prize in Chemistry in 1980.

Berg's investigations led to the birth of a new technology referred to as genetic engineering or gene manipulation.

A practical application of this was the manufacture of insulin from bacterial as distinct from animal sources which had been the practice since the discovery by Banting in 1921.

Berg, was born in Brooklyn New York, a tough neighbourhood which has produced world heavyweight boxing champions including Floyd Patterson and, in more recent years, "Iron" Mike Tyson.

Berg had Russian–Jewish ancestry. His father was a clothing manufacturer. Berg attended local schools before graduating with a Science degree in biochemistry from Penn State University, then a PhD from Case Western Reserve University in 1952. The following seven years were a period of intensive research in various centres including Washington University School of Medicine and Cambridge before starting his tenure at Stanford University in 1959.

During the 1950s he was consumed by the structure of proteins. His childhood interest in science had turned to a preoccupation with how amino acids which are the building blocks of proteins are linked together in a pattern (template) carried within a nucleic acid called messenger RNA.

The many characteristics of life in living creatures, be they small like bacteria, or large like animals and humans, are the result of complicated chemical reactions which are carried out inside a living cell. These chemical reactions all depend on what can be thought of as a chemical machine which exists inside the cell in tiny bodies called chromosomes. The name of this chemical machine is DNA (deoxyribonucleic acid.)

Berg experimented with combining genetic material from different species and a remarkable accomplishment during this period was a method he devised for "cutting" genes, then joining one of these pieces to another piece which had been cut from a different gene. Building upon the findings of Griffith and Avery that genetic material could still transmit the information it carried after it had been boiled, he harnessed a team of brilliant scientists to combine genetic material from different organisms. The fact that this was accomplished in test tubes didn't fool the brilliant researcher for a moment. He knew that he had, in fact, achieved a unique biological phenomenon – artificially. The combination of the two unrelated sources ("father" and "mother") was in fact *reproduction achieved through recombination.*

The word which they used and which is now permanently embedded in scientific lexicon is *recombinant.*

The final piece of the puzzle was actually the work of one of Berg's younger associates called Janet Mertz, a graduate student who had joined his team in the winter of 1970. And the scientist who had provided her with the essential reagent to complete her experiments was none other than Herb Boyer.

Amongst Berg's many talents which become obvious on even a cursory reading of his scientific accomplishments is his capacity for getting the best out of people including those much younger than himself.

The groundbreaking research which took place in the winter of 1970 eventually resulted in the use of this technique to produce the "new" insulin.

It was the use of recombinant technology that resulted in the eventual freedom of Insulin from its age–old dependence on animal sources. Insulin was just one of its many triumphs. Whereas after its discovery in 1921 the next step had been its development followed by delivery to the desperately needy, the modern insulin before delivery was subjected to several more steps. This insulin, by the time it was injected into the patient, had been studied in such minute detail that one could almost say that every one of its molecules had been unravelled, dissected, diced and divided.

Welcome to the New World of science, genetics, biology, medicine, biotechnology and bioethics.

More than once when preparing this monograph and having to familiarise myself with the new language of biotechnology I had to remind myself that in 1971, the year when Berg and Jackson created the first recombinant DNA molecule, the word *biotechnology* had not made it into the Oxford dictionary.

(Karol Ereky (1878-1952), a graduate of the Technical University of Budapest had worked as an agricultural engineer in Hungary. He coined the term "biotechnology" and is regarded by many as the father of biotechnology.)

So if you, gentle reader, have struggled with this section of the narrative, be patient. Some of it was new to me too. You could even skip these parts and move beyond them because the story becomes more interesting before it ends.

Should you decide to do that go to the next chapter.

The Asilomar Conference

Before proceeding to the final chapter in the insulin story it is worth describing the early years of apprehension, anxieties, questions and controversies over the use of recombinant technology which showed that Paul Berg was also a leader of men. The wider implications of his work had not escaped him. All of a sudden, moving genes between the bacterial and the animal world was no longer the stuff of science fiction. If genes could be manipulated in a test tube and the hybrids propagated in living organisms then could not the same be done in "the whole universe of biology with a kind of experimental audacity that was unimaginable in the past?" asked Berg (as quoted by Mukherjee in *The Gene An Intimate History.)*

Mukherjee went on to observe that every field of biology was transformed by the gene-cloning and gene–sequencing technology.

The period immediately after Berg's discovery was marked as much by excitement in scientific circles as by concerns about its biohazards.

A few months after completing his experiments in the summer of 1972 Paul Berg travelled to Erice, a small town on the West Coast of Sicily. He was there to give a talk at a seminar to an audience composed largely of university students from Europe. Berg kept the tone informal and presented his findings in his usual low-key fashion. Remember he was an experienced university lecturer and tutor and had clearly guessed the effect his findings were going to have.

He wasn't wrong.

"The students were electrified," wrote Mukherjee. In addition to the bio hazards which had troubled the scientists, the students raised wider issues about possible effects of genetic engineering in humans including behaviour control. They were excited about the possibility of curing genetic disease but at the same time concerned about scientific intervention to change basic/natural characteristics such as height, colouring and intelligence in humans.

Two conferences of scientists arranged by Berg in January 1973 and in the summer of that year did little to resolve the ethical issues.

In February 1975 Berg, with four other colleagues, organised a conference to which, in addition to scientists, they invited lawyers, journalists and writers.

The site of the conference was Asilomar on the Monterey Peninsula, about an hour's drive out of San Francisco. The area has, over the years, gained publicity through its association with sports stars and artists. Clint Eastwood was elected Mayor of Carmel-by-the Sea in 1986 and the golf course at Pebble Beach is remembered for Tiger Woods blitzing the field to win the 2000 US Open by 15 strokes.

Berg opened the meeting largely to outline the wide-ranging issues which needed to be addressed. The scientists were clear about their concerns but there was little agreement among them.

As seems to be common in today's litigious society it was only when five attorneys took the stage and outlined the legal minefields this scientific advance had created that there was interest in the group of scientists.

The lawyers outlined the legal ramifications of just a single member of a laboratory being infected by a recombinant organism. This could lead to a complete shutdown of the entire institution to say nothing of the spectre of public outcry and the nirvana for activists.

There was stunned silence. You could hear a pin drop.

All whispered conversations, an irritating but common habit, ceased. Research workers, and university professors were suddenly jolted from their closeted academic environments to the tough, uncompromising "winner–take–all" world of commersialism and – especially for lawyers –the fertile field of litigation.

The meeting concluded with five scientists including Berg drafting a plan for the future which stressed caution and proposed a scheme to rank the risk potentials of various genetically changed organisms.

In the final analysis although this conference had addressed, at least partly, the biological risks it had not come to grips with the ethical and moral issues which continue to be a thorn in the side of workers in this remarkable scientific breakthrough of our time.

Thus genes, which had defied scientific scrutiny since the beginning of creation, when at last exposed, turned out to be not so much the servant but the master. The gene which started as the subject of this study turned out to be the teacher interrogating the scientist/student.

It would be impertinent to repeat the cliche about "the genie being let out of the bottle."

MODERN INSULIN DELIVERED

The commercial vehicle for large-scale development of modern insulin was a quintessentially American financial device commonly referred to as venture capitalism. Its earlier name of "development capital" which provided help to smaller entrepreneurial business in the US is perhaps a more easily understood term for what is now a leading source of finance especially for larger ventures.

In the 1970s and 80s around the time modern insulin was creating waves in scientific circles venture capital was gaining momentum as an important, if not the major, source of capital for emerging companies. One of the companies given the forbidden fruit now occupies a place of its own in today's commercial world and in today's lexicon, Apple.

In retrospect the emergence of venture capitalism at that particular time is puzzling because of the general atmosphere of gloom in the United States. It was the time of the Arab oil embargo and the time when the United States had had to swallow the bitter pill of defeat in the war in Vietnam.

Robert Swanson (1947–1999)

"I enjoyed people more than things."

Robert Swanson was, like Paul Berg, born in Brooklyn to a working class family. His father was a shift worker in an aeroplane electrical maintenance team. Swanson was repeatedly reminded during his early years that his generation would be better than the previous generation in his family. He was encouraged to aim for higher education and was the first in his family to graduate with a college degree.

The Massachusetts Institute of technology was for other members of the family an unreachable goal but much to his parents surprise and pride, Swanson was accepted into that institution in 1965. Although he graduated with a degree in chemistry, a summer job in a chemical factory made him realise that he had a particular gift. He could work with people, even difficult ones. He sought a temporary release from MIT to attend the Alfred Sloan School of Management and did a Masters degree. Swanson graduated from MIT in 1970 with a Bachelors degree in Chemistry and Master of Science in Management.

His first contact with genetic recombination project was during his time at a venture capital firm called Kleiner and Perkins which he had joined at the invitation of the firm's founder Eugene Kleiner. However the association was short-lived because of the firm's financial difficulties and in 1975 Swanson was out of a job. But not out of ideas!

He had heard of a new technology, "recombinant DNA". The fact that he was highly unlikely to have understood even the basics of the process did not put him off at all.

Somehow Swanson found a handbook which had been handed out at the Asilomar meeting. In it was a list of the more prominent scientists engaged in the recombinant experiments.

Swanson had little, if any idea of even the basics involved in studying and working with genes.

He decided to employ the technique and tactics with which he was familiar. Cold calls.

Having clearly recognised the importance and prominence of Paul Berg, the optimistic Swanson phoned him. What he did not know was Berg's singular lack of interest in financial gain nor the scientist's concern and respect for the ethics of the technology of which he was a prominent pioneer. The aspiring venture capitalist got short shrift.

Undaunted, Swanson moved on to the next name on the alphabetically compiled list.

Boyer.

Herbert Wayne Boyer (1936 –)

Boyer had come from humble beginnings. He was born in Pennsylvania and had wanted to be a doctor but rejected by the medical school because of poor grades in high school, had to switch to studying microbiology. After gaining a bachelor's degree in biology and chemistry he went on to do a PhD at University of Pittsburgh in 1963. These were his years of taking part in demonstrations in favour of the Civil Rights movement. After three years doing postgraduate work at Yale he had come to San Francisco at the age of 30 as an Assistant Professor at the University of California, San Francisco (UCSF). It was Boyer who had supplied a particular enzyme to Paul Berg's laboratory which had played a significant role in completing the recombinant exercise by Berg's assistant Janet Mertz.

Boyer agreed to meet Swanson for a brief meeting– "a few minutes on Friday afternoon."

He knew nothing about Swanson and had not bothered to check on his credentials. So he was unaware that, without a single exception, every one of Swanson's previous entrepreneurial ventures had failed dismally. Neither did he know that Swanson was unemployed.

Their meeting took place in the Medical Sciences building at University of California San Francisco (UCSF) in January 1976.

Whether Boyer was impressed by Swanson or his idea of starting a company which would use the new discoveries of the potential of genes to be used for making medicines is unclear. What is a matter of record is that the "few minutes" on that Friday afternoon stretched into several hours.

Boyer was impressed by the enthusiasm and drive of the entrepreneur who, at 29, was considerably younger than the academic. Boyer was 40.

Swanson's idea was to start a biotechnology company which would use the recently discovered revolutionary techniques of manipulating bacteria to produce medicines.

There are few greater drivers of initiative and dedication in a medical pursuit than the possibility of relieving or ideally, curing a disease or disability in one's own family. That had happened all over the world following the discovery of insulin in Toronto. The parents of children affected with diabetes were in desperate need of supplies of the insulin extract. Banting couldn't wait to try it on his friend Leonard Thompson. Best had never forgotten his aunt who had died from complications of diabetes.

Boyer's son was suspected of being afflicted with a potential growth disorder. He knew that theoretically it was possible to make Growth hormone in a test tube in his laboratory using a method unknown, at that stage, to all but a few who were working in the field of genetic engineering. Boyer was part of that select group which was capable of making Growth hormone. However he was held back by the understandable hesitation of injecting a bacterial product into his own child. He would much prefer to get something that was manufactured by a reputable pharmaceutical firm and could be purchased with a doctor's prescription and dispensed at a local drug store.

The scientist and university professor Boyer was overridden by Boyer the young man brought up in humble circumstances in Philadelphia. And that young man realised that what he really wanted and needed for his son was a pharmaceutical company. Only this would be a pharmaceutical company with a difference.

It would make medicines not from plants or chemicals but from manipulated genes.

The three–hour meeting ended in a bar where the two men had been sitting for much of the afternoon. They agreed that each of them would put in $500 to pay lawyers to draft the necessary documents required to launch a company.

Swanson went back to his former associate and mentor Eugene Kleiner, now with his own venture firm Kleiner Perkins. Kleiner agreed but only after persuading Swanson to accept $100,000 instead of the half million requested as "seed" money.

In the application to the regulatory body Kleiner had pleaded for approval on the basis of being "in the business of making highly speculative investments."

It worked.

Glancing over one's shoulder at the pursuit of insulin launched by Banting in 1921, it is clear that the hoops to jump through were very different– fewer though perhaps no simpler – from the ones which had to be negotiated before the new team/s could engage in the pursuit of modern insulin.

Genentech A Pioneering Pharmaceutical Biotechnology Company

Genentech, a contraction of **ge**netic **en**gineering **tech**nology, was launched in 1976.

It wrote the names of Swanson and Boyer in the annals of history of commerce and medical science as founders of the world's first pharmaceutical biotechnology company.

Making Insulin, then and now

Fred Banting, a dairy farmer's son had had to go to abattoirs in Toronto to collect the pancreases which had been harvested from cows and pigs, then used methods described by today's scientists as "near–medieval" to make an extract which contained a minuscule amount of insulin. That insulin was not the insulin produced by humans. It was pig and beef insulin.

By contrast Herb Boyer used bacteria, the very nature of which had been altered, "fooled", by mind-boggling scientific manipulations discovered and devised by men like Paul Berg, Herb Boyer and Stanley Cohen, with the potential to produce potentially unlimited quantities of insulin which was structurally and chemically identical to the insulin produced by normal human beings.

Robert Swanson's Drive

If the discovery, development and delivery of insulin in 1921-22 can be attributed to the unceasing efforts and drive of one man, that would be Frederick Banting. Similarly, bringing human insulin from the laboratory and test tube to the bedside of patients was largely driven by the irrepressible and ever–optimistic Robert Swanson.

Boyer and Swanson's first thought as far as the product to be manufactured was insulin. Perhaps they were aware of the stories of the stampede for insulin by patients, parents of children afflicted with the condition, and by physicians at the time of the discovery in 1921.

However, like the Nobel laureate Dorothy Hodgkin, Boyer was hesitant to tackle insulin for the same reason which had made Hodgkin defer the exercise for 16 years. It was the size and complexity of the insulin molecule.

Swanson's knowledge of molecular chemistry was, to all intents and purposes, nil. To him the attraction of producing insulin was its almost unlimited market potential. As Genentech's attorney Tom Kylie was to observe years later, it was "Mr Swanson proposing to make dollars out of DNA."

To temper Swanson's "bull–at–the–gate" approach Boyer had to explain the reason for his apprehension.

Insulin is a large molecule, often referred to as a "macro molecule."

Also called "The Everest of molecules," it is made up of 51 building blocks (amino acids). The large number is perhaps the reason for nature deciding that the hormone was best arranged in not one but two chains, 30 building blocks in one and 21 in the other. Then the two chains had to be joined in a specific position between a building block in one chain to a particular building block in the other. Even the joining was critical because as mentioned earlier any change in these steps made the molecule completely ineffective.

By contrast Somatostatin, also a hormone like insulin was much smaller with only 14 amino acids (building blocks), all in a single chain. Unlike insulin, somatostatin had little market potential. Boyer patiently explained to the impatient Swanson that starting with somatostatin would help them iron out at least some of the technical difficulties before attempting to make insulin.

Swanson was not convinced. He either didn't understand or didn't want to understand because for him the main goal – and prize, was insulin. Still, he bowed to Boyer because the scientist was after all, the one who was going to do the work.

Boyer recruited two more scientists who were experienced in DNA synthesis. Art Riggs and Keiichi Itakura both from the City of Hope hospital in Los Angeles were well known in the small circle of "whip-smart" researchers.

Also at this time Swanson made a choice which was to have an important and long lasting effect on Genentech. He hired an attorney called Tom Kiley. He wanted Kiley to make sure that Genentech's agreements with UCSF and City of Hope hospital were legally sound.

Kiley, in an interview years later admitted that he had absolutely no familiarity with the scientific aspects of the company's work. He didn't even know what *molecular biology* actually stood for.

"Why then did you take the job?" asked the interviewer.

"I just liked the guy," Kiley answered.

Their friendship was to last for the rest of their lives. Kiley, who later joined the company was to play a pivotal role in the development of Genentech and later, crucial legal battles over patent issues involving Genentech and, wait for it, Lilly company. Yes, the original company which had enjoyed a financial bonanza with the Toronto insulin was still a world leader in the marketing of pharmaceuticals including insulin.

Both Boyer and Swanson were also acutely aware that they had strong competition in the race to make insulin. At Harvard University Walter Gilbert, the DNA chemist who later shared the 1980 Nobel Prize for Chemistry with Berg and Sanger had a strong team of scientists working on the same project. A third team in pursuit of the the same goal was busy in UCSF.

Frantic and unrelenting hours of work in the summer of 1977 showed promising signs and in June Boyer and Swanson were told by Riggs and Itakura that they had succeeded in making somatostatin.

Boyer and Swanson flew to Los Angeles to watch the demonstration of the first constructed molecule of somatostatin. The machinery includes detectors of molecules on a sound recorder and also a printout which records the presence of the protein, in this case the hormone Somatostatin. The small group gathered in the laboratory the next morning. The molecular detectors for the presence of somatostatin in the bacteria were turned on. The hush of expectation as the group collectively held its breath waiting for the sound recorder – Swanson was conspicuously agitated – was answered by stubborn silence from the detector. Failure.

Students of history on this subject will not have failed to notice the echo in this incident with that in the pursuit of insulin by Banting when the first injection of his extract had met with the same result – 55 years earlier.

Bob Swanson developed severè chest pain the next day and was rushed to Emergency at the nearest hospital. Fortunately it turned out to be a case of indigestion rather than coronary artery occlusion which the group had feared.

The research group sat down to go through the entire exercise in search of where they might have gone wrong. Checking, rechecking, repeating, arguing, returning to previous references are all bread-and-butter activities of research scientists of which the man in the street has little idea.

Boyer remained with them lending his experience of working with bacteria for over a decade.

It took another three months of intensive work which included suggestions by Boyer before they were ready to try once again. This time, in August 1977, Itakura, who like the other scientists, had been drawn to Swanson's passion for the project, addressed him directly.

"Somatostatin is here."

The Modern Insulin : Assault, Conquest, and Delivery

"I'll attack insulin."

John Jacob Abel 1922.

This time Swanson was not to be denied. He was nothing if not driven. The goal was, and always had been, insulin.

It is an interesting coincidence that the word used by Genentech scientists was the same as the one used by Abel when the Johns Hopkins pharmacologist had decided to work on insulin soon after its discovery in Toronto in 1921. Attack.

Fortunately for the Swanson–Boyer team, fate favoured the entrepreneur. The three months lost after the first failure of efforts to synthesise somatostatin had given their competitors a definite edge. There were rumours that Gilbert's team were on the verge of producing insulin on a large scale. Worse still, the UCSF scientists claimed to have synthesised a small quantity of insulin which was going to be injected into patients.

Swanson didn't actually say so but Boyer had not forgotten his partner's lack of enthusiasm for the somatostatin "diversion". Also concerning was a worsening in Swanson's physical state dominated by increasingly frequent attacks of chest pain which the scientists hoped was still due to indigestion.

Where Genentech had an edge over its rivals especially Gilbert's group in Harvard was the nature of the material being used to make insulin. Gilbert's experiments used the human gene which he introduced into bacteria and which in turn produced insulin. Berg's conferences at Asilomar had culminated in Federal restrictions on the use of recombinant technology in government–funded institutions like Harvard. Gilbert, because he was using the *human* gene which in his experiments was then introduced into bacteria to make insulin would not be permitted to proceed as he had planned. Genentech on the other hand, had *made* the insulin gene in the laboratory, building–block by building–block.

Furthermore, Genentech was a privately funded company not dependent on federal financial support and therefore, possibly, on the government's stipulations.

Simply stated, Genentech made insulin DNA and then put it (the synthetic DNA) into bacteria which then produced "human" insulin – the modern insulin.

With this breakthrough it was "all systems go" as far as Swanson was concerned.

The cramped quarters were no longer adequate. Swanson went on a hunt again.

In early 1978, he found a more substantial building, actually a warehouse, in the south of San Francisco. Unlike the "booth" in San Francisco, the warehouse provided 10,000 square ft. for Genentech's laboratory.

Mukherjee, with an eye and ear for interesting details, wrote that Genentech occupied the front-half of the premises while the back half of the warehouse housed a storage facility for a distributor of porn videos. Clearly there were no limits to Swanson's enterprising approach.

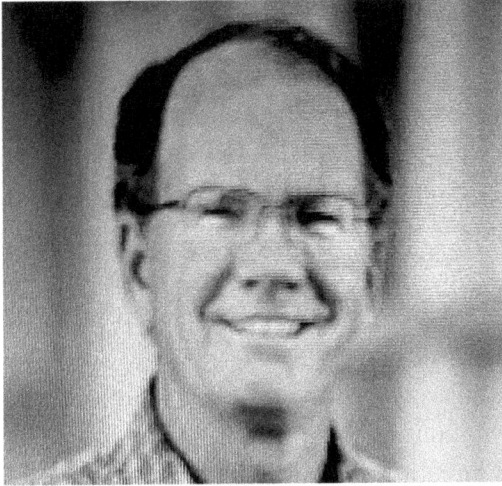

David Goeddel made insulin in a test tube 1978.

In the meantime Boyer expanded their workforce by adding more scientists to Genentech's personnel. One of these scientists was David Goeddel. Even a brief acquaintance with Goeddel would have made one think that he had been hand-picked not by Boyer but by Swanson. The 27-year old's drive and competitive work ethic reminded the venture capitalist of his own attitude to any challenge.

Goeddell was thoroughly familiar with the techniques and traps of cloning. He favoured casual work attire and usually wore sneakers and a black T-shirt emblazoned with the slogan "clone or die." He possessed limitless energy and an infectious enthusiasm.

Now Genentech, with suitably sized premises and a better workforce made human insulin the all consuming goal for the entire group.

Swanson walked around marshalling the troops with cliches like "fortune favours the brave" which drove some of the research scientists crazy simply because none of them needed encouragement. In fact some of the scientists were irritated by the businessman but fortunately Swanson also had an endearing quality to his annoying persistence. They all understood the urgency of making insulin before their competitors.

Perhaps Swanson was right and fortune did favour the brave because, as it turned out, their competitors had troubles of their own. Harvard's Gilbert was trying to bypass the constraints imposed by the government along the lines of the Asilomar recommendations by sending several members of his staff to a facility he had managed to access in England. The UCSF team dispatched a scientist to a pharmaceutical facility in France.

Swanson could hardly contain his delight.

Genentech, unfettered by such handicaps and, in spite of its comparatively smaller size, made spectacular progress.

Mukherjee described the comparison between the nimble, smaller Genentech and the academic behemoth Harvard as "an inverted fable: an academic Goliath versus a pharmaceutical David, one lumbering, powerful, handicapped by size, the other nimble, quick, adept at dancing around rules."

The crucial steps which culminated in the creation of the first batch of recombinant insulin can be summarised as follows:

1. By early summer, in May 1978, the Genentech team had made the two chains of insulin in bacteria.
2. By July, the proteins had been separated, and "purified", from the bacteria in which they had been formed.
3. In early August, proteins which were part of the bacteria were removed, "snipped off" in the jargon of the scientists.
4. Then at last came the culmination of weeks of unceasing work, tension, frustrations and failures.

For step 5, let's imagine for a moment that this historic event was being watched by a fly on the wall. Or perhaps the spirit of the chronic insomniac Bob Swanson ?

David Goeddell was accustomed to working late. It was said that he did not wear a watch. Nor did he have a clock in his laboratory.

Near midnight on August 21, 1978 David Goeddell etched his own name in the insulin story, and took that "one small step for man..."

He joined the two chains of protein which had been created in bacteria and produced the world's first molecule of recombinant insulin.

There is another interesting difference between the discovery in Toronto in the summer of 1921 and the events of 1976 which we have just witnessed.

Whereas in 1921-22, in spite of some internal squabbles over patent rights by men who knew little about it, in the case of modern insulin, Swanson had foreseen the need for the next step at an early stage of the research. He had hired Tom Kiley the attorney for just this part of the exercise.

Therefore it is not surprising that within two weeks of Goeddell making the first molecule of recombinant insulin Genentech applied for a patent for manufacturing insulin.

Unlike the original discovery of insulin the modern insulin fell in the category of an invention. Legislation in the United States through the United States Patents Act specified four categories of inventions which could be patented. These were methods, manufactured materials, machines and compositions of matter. In commercial jargon they were referred to as the "four Ms"

Genentech's attorney, Kiley neatly sidestepped the "four Ms" specified by the Patent's Act and, for the first time in the history of that area of federal administration, applied for a patent for a "DNA vehicle" which was needed to place a gene inside a bacterial cell.

Physicians, scientists and especially men, women and children suffering from diabetes would regard August 21, 1978 as a historic date when human insulin was made artificially but as far as Robert Swanson was concerned the important date was October 26, 1982 because that is when the US Patent and Trademark Office (USPTO) issued to Genentech a patent to use recombinant DNA to produce a protein – such as insulin and, Genentech's first "trial" product, somatostatin.

Genentech lost no time in claiming a prime position in the American stock market as one of the most spectacular "stars in the ascendant" through the meteoric rise of its share price. It is not surprising that given its conspicuously lucrative product (insulin) there would be competition including, at a later stage, bitter court battles over patents. However those are stories for another day. Suffice it to say that Swanson's dream was fulfilled as Genentech went on to produce and market several medical/hormonal products and vaccines including growth hormone.

In 1990 he and Boyer sold to Roche Pharmaceuticals a majority stake in Genentech for $2.1 billion dollars. The following year both Swanson and Boyer stepped down from their positions of CEO and Vice President respectively.

Swanson died from a brain tumor in 1999 aged 52. He had lived in Hillsborough, a suburb situated close to the laboratories of his brainchild Genentech.

That insulin occupies a central, even unique position in the evolution of the biotechnology industry is part of the history of medical and scientific advances. Together with clotting factors for haemophilia, insulin is the first medicine to be created by genetic engineering.

Recombinant DNA technology has enabled modifications to the human insulin molecule. This has led to the development of a new range of insulin preparations with different durations of action including long–acting insulin analoguess such as insulin glargine.

A drawback of insulin production by recombinant technology is the cost, especially in countries where the cost of medical care is borne directly by patients and their relatives.

An indirect consequence of the improvements achieved by the discovery and development of recombinant technology has been research in other directions aimed at improving the care of the diabetic individual. Significant improvements in advances have resulted in preparations seeking to avoid injections of insulin altogether. Insulin preparations which may be inhaled or applied topically have so far not achieved consistent results but research in such areas continues. Automated Delivery systems for insulin have made remarkable progress freeing patients from the need to inject insulin. Once again, at this stage, cost remains a major deterrent.

The pioneering research leading to the discovery and development of recombinant technology by men including Paul Berg, Stanley Cohen, Herb Boyer, their associates and a host of others has changed for ever the research landscape and indeed the future of many areas of chemistry and related branches of study.

There are interesting similarities and differences between the men and women involved in the discovery of insulin in 1921 and those we have met in the story of what I have called the modern insulin which has astounded the scientific world and given new hope to millions of diabetics around the world.

The Future

Reasons for Hope and Optimism

Insulin saved lives.

It transformed the the future of millions of children and adults who had suffered from its deficiency. Many of the men and women so rescued made life–changing contributions to society.

But insulin is a treatment, not a cure for diabetes. Frederick Banting reminded his audience of this in the Nobel lecture he delivered to the dignitaries and to Swedish royalty in 1923.

In 2021, one hundred years after the discovery of insulin in Toronto, diabetes continues to defy all attempts to halt its march and remains one of the fastest growing health challenges of the 21st-century. The number of diabetic adults has tripled over the previous 20 years.

Today diabetes afflicts some 415 million men and women, which equates to one in eleven adults.

It is prevention and prevention alone which will provide relief from this condition.

Frederick Banting's reminder is as pertinent today as it was on that day in 1923.

The remarkable advances made during the research which culminated in the synthesis of modern insulin holds the promise of further advances and give us reasons for hope and optimism. It is appropriate to conclude this account with an illustration of the potential and promise of one such advance.

When Frederick Sanger revealed to the world of molecular chemistry the complete sequence of the amino acids in the insulin molecule what was admired and appreciated by his fellow scientists but perhaps not by the man in the street was the long period of sustained effort expended by the quiet, self-deprecating scientist. Even today many may not know that Sanger's solo labour had occupied 12 years of work at the laboratory bench.

And this is where the remarkable advances which have been referred to earlier need to be recognised.

Whereas Sanger took 12 years to work out the sequence in his project on insulin, modern advances in technology have achieved such great improvements in the design of scientific instruments that Sanger's manual techniques can now be replicated far more rapidly through automation.

Furthermore, technological advances have provided the dual advantage of faster sequencing at a lower cost.

The latest techniques in what is now referred to as next generation genome sequencing (NGS) have taken scientific accomplishment to dizzying heights. These newer methods for which the scientists have been honoured, now enable researchers to read the human genome one million times faster and at a fraction of the cost of the earlier technologies.

Comparing recent and current advances with the situation in earlier times when it used to take ten years and $3 billion to read the first human genome leaves one speechless because today's machines can perform the same task in one hour at a cost of $1000.

Like many who have featured in this story, selfless men and women continue to strive to improve the lot of suffering mankind all around the world.

That, I believe, is a reason to embrace hope and expectation with optimism.

POSTSCRIPT

Shankar Balasubramaniam and David Klenerman of Cambridge University shared the biennial 2020 Millennium Technology Prize of €2 million with Pascal Mayer, the founder of the French firm Alphanosos, for creating next–generation genome sequencing, NGS.

The announcement was delayed because of the Covid–19 pandemic.

It is pertinent to acknowledge that the technology will assist in determining the complete DNA sequence of an organism which may prove to be crucial in the battle against the Covid–19 pandemic.

Did I say sequencing?

The late Fred Sanger would have smiled.

THE END

SMALL STEPS: A BRIEF HISTORICAL CHRONOLOGY OF INSULIN

"Little drops of water,
Little grams of sand,
Make the mighty ocean."

From *Little Things*, 1845 by Julia Abigail Carney from "Poet's Corner" in the Boston Trumpet.

2650BC: Emhotep, physician and advisor to the pharaoh Djoser describes excessive passage of urine as a sign of diabetes.
Nearly 3000 years pass before the next epoch of Greek and Roman knowledge adds to information on diabetes.
Second century BC: Ebers papyrus, recorded diabetes and its treatment with medical recipes including incantations and concoctions. They were published by their discoverer and owner George Ebers in 1875.
125-199 A.D.: Claudius Galenus ("Galen") calls diabetes "diarrhoea urinosa." Diabetes is said to be a transliteration of the Greek word which means "passing through" or "siphon".
150 A.D. Aretaeus of Cappadocia writes a detailed description of diabetes.
400–500 A.D. The Indian physician Sushruta and surgeon Charaka define diabetes is *madhumeha w*hich means "honey urine."

980–1037 A.D. Date of the birth and death of the Persian physician Avecenna who described excessive appetite and gangrene as part of the clinical picture of diabetes.

1674: The Oxford Professor Thomas Willis after tasting sweetness in the urine of a patient with diabetes introduces the term diabetes mellitus.

1776: Matthew Dobson demonstrated brown crystals after evaporating urine of a patient and called the crystals "brown sugar".

1788: an Englishman called Cawley reported post-mortem findings in one case which showed a shrivelled pancreas which contains stones but did not comment on the possible role of the pancreas in causing diabetes.

1797: Englishman John Rollo measured sugar in the urine of a glycosuric and wrote a book on the subject.

1869: Paul Langerhans, a medical student describes the islets of Langerhans.

1875: Apollinaire Bouchardat writes (in French) one of the earliest textbooks on diabetes, *De la Glycosuria ou Diabete Sucre.*

1876: Birth of James Macleod, part of the original insulin team.

1889: Oscar Minkowski demonstrates the pancreas as the "seat" of diabetes.

1891: Birth of Frederick Banting, the discoverer of insulin.

1892: Birth of James Bertram Collip, part of the original insulin team.

1898: Bernhard Naunyn publishes *Der Diabetes Melltus (sic).*

1899: Birth of Charles Herbert Best, Banting's assistant.

1910: Edward Sharpy Schafer suggests "insulin" as the name for the missing secretion of the pancreas responsible for diabetes.

1913: Francis Madison Allen publishes *Glycosuria and Diabetes.*

1916: Elliott P. Joslin writes the first English language textbook on diabetes, *The Treatment of Diabetes Mellitus.* It is published by Lea & Febiger of Philadelphia and New York.

1918: Elliott P. Joslin publishes the first English language instruction manual for patients with diabetes.

1921: Insulin discovered by Banting and Best in Toronto.

1922: First successful insulin injection given to a patient with diabetes in Toronto.

1923: Insulin developed by pharmaceutical firm Lilly of Indianapolis, USA.

1923: Nobel Prize awarded to Banting and Macleod.

1925: Insulin crystals from bovine pancreas demonstrated by John Jacob Abel aged 68.

1936: Protein Zinc Insulin, (PZI) developed by Hans Christian Hagedorn of Denmark.

1939: Globin insulin, a medium–duration preparation is marketed in Europe.

1940: Frederick Banting dies in a plane crash.

1950: Neutral Protamine Hagedorn (NPH) insulin becomes a "best seller."

1951: Lente insulin competes with NPH.

1955: Frederick Sanger demonstrates structure of insulin.

1960: Rosalyn Yalow describes radioimmunoassay of insulin.

1967: Donald Steiner describes proinsulin.

1972: Paul Berg discovers and names recombinant DNA.

1976: Genentech launched by Robert Swanson and Herb Boyer.

1978: David Goeddel synthesises the first recombinant Insulin molecule.

1982: US Patent and Trademark Office (USPTO) issues patent to Genentech to produce recombinant insulin.

1982: Humulin developed by Genentech is licensed to Eli Lilly and becomes the first marketable insulin created through recombinant DNA technology. It was the first recombinant pharmaceutical product approved for use in the USA.

1990: Insulin pen devices introduced for use by patients to inject insulin.

Currently, insulin-delivery devices using sophisticated technologies enable patients to monitor their glucose levels and have appropriate (predetermined) amounts of insulin delivered directly into the bloodstream without the need for injections.

1991: Swanson and Boyer leave Genentech after selling a majority stake in Genentech to Roche.
1996: Short-acting insulin analogue added to the range of preparations available for patients with diabetes.
1999: Genentech founder Robert Swanson dies aged 52.

2001: Long–acting insulin analogue added to the range of preparations available for clinical use heralding more convenient forms of insulin.

2020: Millennium Technology Prize awarded for genome sequencing.

ACKNOWLEDGEMENTS

It was during a visit to the Joslin Diabetes Centre in 2014 when I saw and was fascinated by the amount of material which had been collected for preservation and historic importance as well as a tribute to the founder Dr. Elliott Proctor Joslin (1869–1962). Dr Donald M. Barnett had voluntarily come out of retirement to help with this project and I wish to, once again, record my gratitude and appreciation for Don's generosity in giving me access to the material held in the archives. Don was engaged in writing about Dr Joslin's life but unfortunately was interrupted by unforeseen health issues. I remain indebted to Dr Donald Barnett, Matt Brown the Joslin Archivist as well as the CEO at the time, Mr John Brooks for giving me access to the material and sending me copies of documents and photographs in the succeeding years mainly for my book *Joslin A Pioneer in Diabetes Care* which was published in 2019. Some of the material from it is repeated in this work.

The 1st edition of the Joslin textbook, *Treatment of Diabetes Mellitus* by Elliott P. Joslin and published by Lee and Febiger in 1916 was consulted for information on the treatment of diabetes up to that time. This was long before Insulin was discovered.

It had taken me several years to obtain this much-valued book and I wish to acknowledge the help and generosity of my friend and colleague Professor Milton Roxanas of Sydney University who used his knowledge of medical history and his knack for finding rare books to discover the first edition of the Joslin text.

The third edition of the textbook was consulted for an essay on the early history of diabetes during the period immediately following the discovery of insulin by Banting and Best in Toronto, Canada.

The early editions of the instruction manual for patients, *A Diabetic Manual For The Mutual Use Of Doctor And Patient by Elliott P. Joslin,* first published by Lea and Febiger in 1918 was used for information on instructions provided to patients before the discovery of insulin.

Joslin's Diabetes Mellitus, 13th edition edited by Kahn and Weir published by Lea and Febiger and Joslin's Diabetes Mellitus, 14th edition edited by Kahn, Weir, King, Jacobson, Moses and Smith and published by Lippincott Williams & Wilkins were consulted for the timelines of significant discoveries in diabetes.

Elliott P. Joslin, MD: A Centennial Portrait by Donald M. Barnett, MD provided material for Joslin's comments on the epidemic of diabetes.

Books by Michael Bliss: *The Discovery of Insulin.*
William Osler A Life in Medicine.
Harvey Cushing A Life in Surgery.

Henry B.M. Best: *Margaret and Charley the personal story of Dr. Charles Best, the Co-Discoverer of Insulin* published by The Dundurn Group Toronto - Oxford.

Siddhartha Mukherjee: *The Gene. An Intimate History.*

Many sources have been acknowledged in the book where I have used their material.

Professor Munichoodappa, a lifelong friend and colleague was extremely enthusiastic and encouraging when I discussed writing this book. Professor Suresh Mehtalia also an ex-Joslin Fellow remains a close friend who encouraged my work on the history of diabetes in general and insulin in particular.

Vijendra Kumar and I were 12 and 13-year-olds in a boarding school in Fiji. He pursued a distinguished career as a journalist and then as the Editor-in – Chief of one of the more influential publications in the South Pacific, *The Fiji Times*. Vijendra is remembered and held in esteem for his remarkable insight, commonsense and humility. In him I always found not only a willing listener but also a source of sound advice and information on various subjects I have covered in this book. Vijendra read the manuscript and made several constructive suggestions.

Professor Eberhard Standl, a close friend since our Joslin days also read the manuscript and made several helpful suggestions especially relating to current views on various aspects of diabetes. Eberhard also sent me the photograph of Georg Ebers which is included in Part 1 of this book.

The Osler Society: Professors Milton Roxanas and Rolando del Maestro and Mr. Richard Osborn have been mentioned in the text. Milton has been especially generous with not only information but support and encouragement throughout this project.

Mr Richard Osborn, the librarian of the Osler Library in London located a recorded copy of the Osler Oration given by Charles Best in London in 1957. He then found a sound-technician with expertise in such matters to convert the recording to a sound file which was then emailed to me. I'm deeply grateful to Mr Osborn for all the trouble he took to do so and once again to Milton Roxanas for putting me in touch with Richard.

Cheryl Fleming, with typical generosity and willingness, typed The Osler Oration from the sound files.

Michael Lockwood, a wizard of photography, helped me with images for the text and cover.

Tilak Sinha solved computer-related and formatting issues.

Finally, as always, I thank Lee for reading the manuscript, designing the cover and for her patience in listening to my endless stories over the months spent on the preparation of this work.

All errors and omissions are mine and I offer sincere apologies for each one.

Shailendra K. Sinha
Sydney
Australia
March 2022

INDEX

Naunyn B, 20,158
Noble EC, 35,109,160
Noorden CV,158
Osborn R, 220,321
Osler EB, 150
Osler, oration 220
Osler W,3,253
Paget J,70
Pasteur L, 5,149
Paulescu NC,189,200,202
Pauling L,268
Pedersen H,177
Pedersen T,177
Petersen A,176
Pratt JH,vi
Putnam F,128
Rabinowich D,169
Recklinghausen FV, 252
Riggs A,260
Roach E, 32,45,196
Robertson DE,155
Robinson W,75
Rollo J, 7
Ross G "Billy" 106
Roux E,149
Roscoe,160
Roxanas M,33,219,321
Ryder T,144
Sanger F,260.261,283
Schumann R, 39
Scott DA, 189,241
Sharpey-Shaeffer E,199
Siegel M,170
Simmons M,27
Sinha T,321
Sprague RG,144
Standl E,321

Starr CL,32,51
Steiner D,261
Swanson R,298,310
Taylor NB,65
Thatcher M,274
Thompson L,100,194
Tory HM,117
Victoria Queen,150
Virchow R, 17,257
Wagner R,39
Walden G 166
Watson J,268
Waugh D,98
Wells HG,144
Whipple G,142
White P xi
Williams JR, 137,179
Willis T,7
Willoughby P,25
Willoughby T,25
Woodyatt R,36, 84,110
Yalow R,261,275

www.ingramcontent.com/pod-product-compliance
Lightning Source LLC
Chambersburg PA
CBHW072048020426
42334CB00017B/1431